The Waiting Game

J MERRILL FORREST

Hashtag PRESS

This edition published in Great Britain by Hashtag Press 2017

Text copyright © Jane Merrill Forrest 2017
Copyright cover design © Mina Bach 2017
Copyright cover photograph © George Panos 2017

The moral right of the author has been asserted

All rights reserved. No part of this publication may be reproduced, stored in retrieval system, or transmitted, in any form or by any means without the prior written permission of the publisher, nor be otherwise circulated in any form of binding or cover other than that in which it is published and without a similar condition being imposed on the subsequent purchaser.

All characters in this publication are fictions and any resemblance to real persons, living or dead, is purely coincidental.

A CIP catalogue for this book is available from the British Library.

ISBN 978-0-9957806-6-8

Typeset in Garamond Classic 11.25/14 by Blaze Typesetting

Printed in Great Britain by Clays Ltd, St Ives plc

HashtagPRESS

HASHTAG PRESS BOOKS
Hashtag Press Ltd
Kent, England, United Kingdom
Email: info@hashtagpress.co.uk
Website: www.hashtagpress.co.uk
Twitter: @hashtag_press

*For George, my husband and my best friend,
who makes all things possible.
For anyone, anywhere, who is working in any capacity
to ease the needs of people with dementia and their loved ones.*

Also by J Merrill Forrest

Flight of the Kingfisher

For the latest news and exclusive material from
J Merrill Forrest visit:
www.jmforrest.com

Acknowledgements:

My heartfelt thanks to Deborah Harrowell, specialist dementia care nurse of many years' experience, who helped me with information about dementia care from the 1980s to the present. If there are any errors they are purely mine. I spoke to many people, who wish not to be named but were willing to share their stories about their experiences with loved ones who suffered from dementia – they know who they are and how much I appreciated their candour when talking about such difficult times.

Thanks also to Inspector Steve McGrath who answered my questions about murder case police procedures. I am grateful to my early-draft readers, Penny Jones, Sue Packer, Jessica Harrowell and my always supportive husband, George Panos, for their honest and helpful feedback.

The cover features a beautiful archway in a private garden, taken by my husband with the kind permission of owner David Hutt.

Finally, I thank Hashtag Press for having faith in me and bringing the book to publication.

Part One

WHERE DO THEY GO?

Chapter 1

ERIN
Dementia Nurse
Derbyshire, 1989

Erin glanced up as Hester, the newest trainee, came into the bathroom with a pile of clean towels that she should have delivered ten minutes ago. Holding back a sigh of exasperation, Erin wondered why the younger woman could not grasp how fast they needed to move if they were to get everyone in their care up, washed, dressed, and into the dining room in time for breakfast. If it came to a competition, Erin thought, she'd have one, probably two patients completely ready before the younger nurse had managed to get just one out of bed.

Erin's slender frame belied a wiry strength, and almost a decade of experience had taught her how to safely and quickly lift people far heavier than she was. She knew that not one of her patients would ever complain about how she treated them, because although she worked at tremendous speed for the whole of her shift, she never showed anything but the utmost care and compassion.

As Erin returned her attention to the patient she was bathing, Hester said, "I think it's such a shame, don't you, to end your days like that? I mean, the ones this far gone have no meaningful life, do they? Doesn't seem right to me to keep them going; I certainly wouldn't want to be left in this state, not knowing who or where I was."

Hardly able to believe her ears, Erin reared up and swivelled on her heels to face Hester, soapy fists on slim hips, fury darkening her grey-blue eyes. "*Keep them going*? How dare you speak like that!" she hissed. She lowered her voice to a fierce whisper, "Just because some of our patients can't communicate and don't physically react to anything doesn't mean they can't hear and understand what's said around them. Honestly, you talk as if they should be put down like sick animals! If you feel like that then you're in the wrong job!"

Hester held her hands up, palms outwards, placating. "I didn't mean anything by it, I'm just saying . . ."

"Well, don't! Don't speak at all if you can't keep thoughts like that to yourself."

Directing a last glare of contempt at Hester, Erin retrieved the sponge from the water and began to soap the patient's back.

"Your daughter is coming to visit today, so we must have you all spruced up. We need to get you looking your best, don't we? Can you sit up a bit for me?"

The man, elderly beyond his years, did not react at all. He sat like a helpless child on the lifting seat in the bathtub, his thin white legs straight out, arms limp, rheumy eyes unfocused. He was totally unresponsive so Erin had no idea whether he was aware of the texture of the sponge or the sharp, citrusy smell of the soap and shampoo or the warmth of the spray of water rinsing him clean.

Did he hear and understand the words of reassurance and general chatter that Erin always kept up with him, as she did with all her patients? The change from when he'd been completely rational to showing only brief periods of lucidity, if that's what they'd been, to this almost trance-like state had been rapid and merciless.

When he'd first arrived as a day patient and then during the early days as a full-time resident, he had looked around with bright-eyed interest, eaten his meals unaided, enjoyed watching the television, joined in some of the activities, and he had loved to chat with staff and fellow residents as well as his visitors. His animated conversation had changed to a repetitive asking of the same questions over and over. Then a couple of weeks ago, from the time he'd been woken up as usual at the start of the day, he'd been completely, utterly absent, as if all signs of him but the purely physical had disappeared overnight.

Since then, all the staff in the care home were waiting to see if he would come back, even if it meant coping with the querulous, endlessly repeating questions again, but Erin was beginning to suspect that the Ralph Maddocks of today would last until he died. It was his family she felt really sorry for; although he was still here in body, they had already lost and were grieving for the relative they'd known and loved so dearly.

Hester, visibly sulking at the telling off, jabbed at the button to bring the bath seat up while Erin held Ralph so he couldn't slip off. She grabbed the towel from the chair and held it ready to wrap around Ralph as soon as he was safely out of the bath and Erin had him standing on the mat. Without a word to Erin, she marched back into the bedroom to strip the sheets from the bed and pile them just inside the door for collection.

In the first few days Hester had insisted on dumping the piles of dirty clothes and linen in the corridor, giving no thought to the residents who could so easily trip over them walking to and from their rooms. That's what truly irritated

Erin, when people didn't give any consideration to how their actions could cause difficulties or even harm to someone else.

"Here we are then, Mr Maddocks." Erin started to gently but briskly rub Ralph dry so he wouldn't get cold. "Goodness, I swear you've lost even more weight since yesterday, you weigh less than a bag of feathers. Let's get your hair dry too, and then we can get you dressed and take you downstairs for breakfast."

Erin guided Ralph into the bedroom and helped him to sit on the narrow bed, which was still awaiting clean sheets, so she could get him dressed. Ralph was soon clothed in his underwear, a white, soft cotton vest, incontinence pants with a fresh pad, and thick beige socks. Erin got his socks on, a job Hester seemed to find almost as difficult as she found putting tights on the female patients, whereas Erin always managed them with no trouble at all.

Meanwhile, Hester laid out his outer clothes on the end of the bed: a pair of dark brown trousers, cream shirt, pale green cardigan and a jaunty red tie. When he'd still been able to look after himself, or ask for what he wanted, Ralph had taken great pride in his appearance.

A member of staff had suggested that he didn't need to wear a tie any more, but Erin felt it important for someone of Ralph's generation, and also for his family to always see him smartly turned out. She insisted that a small selection of his ties remain hanging in his wardrobe, and she had even taken the time to prepare them so one just needed to be placed round his neck, tucked under his collar and the knot tightened. She'd done this to save herself precious seconds, but also because she knew how few of the younger nurses and carers would know how to knot a tie for themselves, let alone do it for someone else.

Well, she had high standards, and no matter how often she

was told to spend less time on her patients, she simply would not comply. They were flesh and blood *people*, for goodness sake, not shop window dummies to be dressed and arranged for the convenience of others!

Erin always had her charges ready on time, and that, surely, was evidence enough that she should be able to carry on as she had always done. She felt deep in her heart that some of the care protocols were misguided at best, plain wrong at worst. Restraint, for instance. When patients got agitated, or wanted simply to walk round in circles, they were often restrained to prevent falls or wandering away, and it distressed Erin to have to do it or watch it being done.

Not long ago, a patient had managed to struggle out of the restraining chair and suffered a broken hip when he'd fallen to the floor. Erin, distressed beyond measure, had said to a senior nurse, "What must it be like to have your perception of the world irrevocably changed as they have? How would we feel if we were prevented from standing up or stretching our legs? There must be a better way." But the nurse, just weeks away from retirement, had disappointed Erin by merely shrugging and replying with no sense of irony that it was for their own safety.

But there were signs of change for the better, and Erin was embracing them with optimism, reading everything she could get her hands on about the research being undertaken. She had chosen as a career what many regarded as a difficult, thankless job, but she had come into it with the mind-set that first and foremost it was the patient's welfare and dignity that mattered. She still felt the same and was pleased to see that the future might be much brighter for those in her profession and, more importantly, those who came into their care.

She used a soft brush to smooth the baby-fine white hair,

then draped a small clean towel round his shoulders while she quickly ran the electric shaver over his cheeks and chin. Finally, she gave the heavy, thick glasses a good clean on her apron and settled them on Ralph's bulbous nose. The whole time she was ministering to him his eyes gazed vacantly downwards.

Erin crouched in front of Ralph so she could adjust the collar of his shirt and straighten the knot of his tie before putting on his comfy, soft leather shoes. Some of the residents always wore slippers, but Ralph had once said with a humorous twinkle in his eye, "Slippers are to be worn with pyjamas and dressing gowns, and nightwear, like nakedness, should only be seen in bedrooms." At Erin's suggestion, his granddaughter had purchased two pairs of leather shoes that fastened with Velcro straps, smart enough to satisfy Ralph, and easy to slip on and off and adjust if his feet swelled, as they sometimes did.

Gazing into his faraway eyes Erin said, "Where are you, Ralph Maddocks? Are you aware of me? Of anything? If nothing else, I hope that you know you're being properly looked after and how much your family loves you."

Ralph's expression did not change, so Erin patted his veined, large-knuckled hands where they rested listlessly on his lap, wishing with all her heart that she could have seen even the merest flicker. A slow blink would be wonderful, or a twitch of the fingers. Anything at all.

But when nothing happened she had to wonder for the thousandth time if Hester could be right. No, not about 'putting them out of their misery,' for who knew if they were miserable? But she simply did not and could not believe that they were nothing more than mindless, empty shells that could only maintain the essentials of breathing, eating, toileting, walking, sleeping and waking up. Surely, somewhere deep inside, they had to have some sense of their surroundings and of being led around and made to sit in that particular chair, eat that food, lie down in that bed? Medical technology could not provide an answer, and maybe never would be able to, but it didn't stop Erin thinking about it constantly.

Not long after his arrival, Ralph had started to believe himself fourteen years old and kept demanding to know when his dad would be home. He wanted to show him the model Spitfire he had made and so carefully painted in camouflage colours, the transfers pasted precisely to match the illustration on the kit box.

When this phase started he, of course, had stopped recognising his daughter or grandchildren because, in the reality his mind had slipped into, he was just a young boy still living with his mum and dad.

Sighing, and wishing again that Ralph would at least come back to that early teenager state when at least you could converse with him, Erin rose from her crouching position, apologising with a laugh as both her knees loudly clicked.

"If I'm like this now," she said. "What am I going to be like in twenty or thirty years' time, eh?"

She gently pulled Ralph up into a standing position then led him by the elbow out of the bedroom, along the corridor, and into the dining room, leaving Hester to clean the bathroom and make the bed.

Ralph was the last of Erin's charges to arrive, so she took charge of feeding him. After draping a cloth round him to protect his clothes, she sat between him and Wilfred, a long-term resident, at the breakfast table.

Wilfred was well into his nineties but like the others sitting round the table, he was capable of feeding himself, so she only needed to keep half an eye on the rest of them while she fed Ralph. As he could not say what he wanted to eat, Erin asked for a bowl of porridge as it was the easiest option, and he'd always enjoyed it when he'd been able to choose for himself.

She tested the temperature before scooping up the first small spoonful, holding Ralph's chin to encourage him to close his mouth, chew and swallow. He took about five mouthfuls, then simply stopped, slack-mouthed, unaware of the milky porridge dribbling down his chin.

Wilfred had finished his toast and asked what time they'd be having breakfast. Erin, while keeping an eye on Ralph, answered him softly, placing herself in his world rather than trying to bring him into the real one.

"Breakfast will be in a little while, Wilfred, so have another piece of toast if you want one, there's plenty on that plate. And you haven't finished that nice of cup of tea, have you?"

Wilfred grinned, showing the few teeth he had left. Another five or ten minutes and he'd be pacing up and down, ten steps one way then turning round and taking ten steps back, asking over and over what time the bus was coming. Or, he would start on his other querulous thread, where he fretted that he had no change to buy a newspaper. But now he poured a little tea from the cup into its matching saucer and blew on it. As he tipped the saucer to his lips and made a noisy show of slurping it down, Erin grinned at him while the others at the table groaned. Ralph, had he been aware of it, would have groaned too at such behaviour.

When it became clear that Ralph would take no more porridge, Erin deftly wiped his mouth, gently admonishing him for not finishing the bowl.

"No wonder you're so skinny, you don't eat enough to feed a bird."

She pushed the bowl away and waited, still hoping against hope that Ralph would show signs of knowing where he was and what was happening. Erin was fond of all the residents in the care home, but she had a bit of a soft spot for this one because he was similar in looks to her grandfather. The resemblance ended there, though, for her grandad had simply dropped dead in his beloved potting shed one day, so hadn't had the misfortune of suffering a lingering end like so many people.

Deciding everyone at her table could be moved to the lounge to wait for their visitors, due to arrive in about an hour's time, Erin looked around at the other residents as she walked through the dining room.

A few knew what day it was and that they were living in a care home, and some lived contentedly in times gone past, singing old songs or chatting to each other as if they were in another era. Some were agitated, angry, crying or fretful and would not be comforted. But a handful seemed completely absent, just like the man shuffling by her side, and she couldn't accept that there was nothing left anywhere of the people they'd once been.

She'd talked about it to other carers, to her husband, mother, sisters and friends, saying, "Some of them are aware of who they are, but not where or when they are. They live in the past because they've been robbed of their memories of their later years, yet they seem content as long as we go into their reality and not keep trying to drag them into ours. It's hard, but you can say that those people are still very much with us. It's the others, the really severe cases who are completely absent that I'm talking about. We just don't know if they see or hear anything; they don't speak, yet their bodies go on functioning.

"Where is the mind, the spirit, the soul, the whatever-it-is that makes us who we are? I can't believe that the essence of someone still living and breathing is just lost for all eternity as if the person never existed. It can't be the same as where we go when we're dead, but they must go somewhere, surely? I just wish I knew!"

Her words and questions led to all sorts of debates, but the discussions mostly ended up being about the complexities of the human brain, not along the esoteric lines Erin was thinking. Most of them did not believe in life after death, or didn't want to spend time thinking about it, nor could they comprehend what she meant when talking about the spirit or soul. No, her questions were far too big, too frightening, for those she talked to, and the only thing her family and friends agreed on was they simply couldn't do the job Erin did. Many asked her why she didn't go into general nursing in a nice big hospital instead.

After a time, she'd learned to keep her thoughts to herself, but when she was looking after Ralph and others like him the big question continued to reverberate in her own mind: *Where do they go?*

Part Two

DEPARTURES

Chapter 2
FINLAY
Scotland, 1991

The silence stretched out as Finlay and his wife struggled to absorb what the consultant had just told them. They'd known. Of course they'd known. But hearing the stark prognosis spoken out loud and realising that this time there was no chance of another remission was still gut-wrenchingly shocking. The consultant's blunt words, though tactfully delivered, seemed to reverberate around the room, getting louder and louder until Fin wanted to put his hands over his ears to shut them out.

His disease had reached the terminal stage, so this was it. This really was it.

Mr Anderson, glancing first at Fin's open medical file, then flicking his gaze from Fin to Aileen and back down to his notes, cleared his throat and said, "Would you like some time alone? Or perhaps we should schedule another appointment to talk about your options?"

Fin gave a bitter laugh. "You mean there are options?"

"Yes, of course there are. But are you sure you're ready to talk things through now? As I say, we can make it another time."

His expression and tone of voice were sympathetic, but his body language betrayed his discomfort and Fin wondered how many conversations like this he had to have on a weekly, perhaps even daily basis. He thought, too, that there were likely other patients out there steeling themselves for their turn in this room. He hoped some of them would go home with better news than that he'd just received.

As if from far away Fin heard Aileen reply that they should discuss everything now so they could make their preparations, but he couldn't concentrate and only caught the occasional, colossal words when he thought about the reality behind the mere sounds coming out of their mouths: chemo, steroids, buying a little more time, pain management, palliative care, hospice.

He concentrated on the consultant's hands, fingers tightly interlaced, resting on top of Fin's own thick medical file. His nails looked well-kept and manicured, quite different to Fin's own chewed nails and ragged cuticles. There was a wide gold band on the finger of his right hand that looked similar to Fin's own wedding ring. Was Mr Anderson married, he wondered, or divorced? A widower? Did he have children? The consultant knew so much about his personal life, but Fin knew virtually nothing about his.

He mentally shook himself; why on earth was he thinking such inconsequential thoughts about Mr Anderson's private life when he was all too soon going to leave his wife a widow, his son fatherless?

He forced himself to concentrate. Aileen held herself erect in her chair, scrubbing the tears away before they could fall unchecked down her face. He could tell from the tone of her voice how tight her throat was, but she was forcing out her questions and insisting on better explanations if she didn't understand the medical terms Mr Anderson had a habit of slipping into.

But even though it was him they were discussing, he couldn't join in the discussion because it was about a future that would be, for him, much too short-lived.

His eyes roamed around the consulting room, so similar to the very many he and Aileen had sat in during the past two years or so. At their third or fourth appointment, he couldn't exactly remember which, they'd sat side by side, just like now, in front of a different specialist, expecting to hear that there was a simple and treatable reason for the persistent pain in his lower back.

They'd listened in mounting disbelief to the explanation of the results of the many tests and scans, and numbly agreed to an exploratory operation under general anaesthetic. Then had followed the post-surgery discussion where they'd met Mr Anderson for the first time, and he'd delivered the mind-numbing revelation that Fin had cancer. Worse, it was aggressive and had already metastasised, but there was a glimmer of hope as long as he could endure the surgery and the gruelling chemotherapy that must follow.

At home later, still reeling from that initial bombshell and the dawning realisation of how bloody hard the treatment would be on both of them, not just himself, he had forced himself to nod and to smile agreement when Aileen had insisted that they could beat the prognosis, that the operation and the treatment regime would work.

Since then, since that first, dreadful night when they'd sat up in bed until the early hours, crying and going over and over what was happening and what was going to happen, how many times had she picked him up when he'd been in danger of sinking into despair? She had even made him laugh once when she'd stood before him, glaring down at the region of his stomach, giving warning to the cancer cells that were every moment dividing and further invading his body that they would be eradicated.

When he'd come round from the anaesthetic after his first operation, she had been there, waiting for him to wake up. She had leaned over so she could lay her head beside his on the pillow and, gently lacing her fingers with his, had whispered, "As long as we pull together, Finlay Kelburn, we can beat this thing. We will beat this thing, for us and for our wee boy."

'For us and our wee boy' had become their mantra.

Recovery had not been as quick as hoped and Fin spent much longer in the hospital than they'd anticipated. His and Aileen's absences from the house were having a detrimental effect on their seven-year-old boy and they were worried about him.

Alex started saying that his Granny Mairi was visiting him in the night. When Fin had sat him on his lap and told him that Granny Mairi had died a long time ago in a car accident with Grampy Donald, before Alex had been born, the little boy had replied, "Oh, I know that, Daddy! She told me. But she says she likes to come and see us, and Grampy is with her sometimes but he never says anything. She's a tiny lady, isn't she?"

Fin hadn't known what to say to that. Yes, his mother had been a tiny lady, and he supposed Alex could see that from a framed photograph that stood on the sideboard, but the lad also seemed to know other things about her that made Fin wonder.

Aileen, on the other hand, was most unhappy about it and said it was more important than they'd realised that Alex be allowed to continue in his usual routine as much as possible. She asked her mother if she would be willing to temporarily move in and look after him and she had readily agreed, enabling

Alex to attend his school, have regular, well-cooked meals, play outside with this friends, or have them round for tea, enjoy fun outings with his Granny and, at weekends his Grampy Muir would join them. It seemed to work, for Alex stopped mentioning Mairi once his other Granny came to look after him.

What Alex couldn't do was visit the hospital, as it was too big a risk that he might bring in an infection, such as a cold. In fact, anyone with an infection of any sort were told they had to keep well away from Fin until they were clear of it, and some people, unable to cope with Fin's illness, had chosen to keep away full stop. So true that one finds out who their real friends are when adversity strikes.

When Fin had at last been allowed to go home, they still had to adjust their lives to the routine of his being a regular hospital outpatient. Aileen insisted on being by his side so he wouldn't endure alone the exhausting rounds of chemotherapy, radiotherapy, scans, blood tests, and pills. So many pills. They did it all together, every step, barely leaving one another's side. Aileen's parents came and went as they were needed, grateful that they could be of genuine help while spending so much precious time with their grandson.

Then came the miracle. Remission.

Aileen had insisted on celebrating that fine summer's day and to Fin it had felt is if they were emerging, blinking and gasping, from a cold and terrible darkness into warm, glittering sunlight. Family and close friends had gathered the following weekend, bringing wine and gifts of the best Scotch whisky and, best of all, loud conversation and laughter, breathing life into the little house that had been quiet and sombre for too long.

Fin had moved among their guests with Alex perched on

his shoulders, laughing and joking as if the whole thing had been nothing more than a bad dream. Aileen had smiled as she offered sandwiches and home-made cakes, smiled as she made pots of tea and coffee, found wine glasses and handed out napkins, smiled as she agreed at how wonderful it all was. But he could see the shadow behind her eyes and knew she couldn't bring herself to believe the ordeal was truly over.

When the pain had returned in the biting cold of the following Scottish winter, even worse than before, the consultant had called them in for a battery of tests straight away. They had not dared say out loud what they suspected those tests would find, and now here they were, having their worst fears confirmed by Mr Anderson.

This is it, Fin said to himself, picturing a timer with his name on it. There was just a little dark sand remaining in the top bulb, trickling inexorably and far too quickly to the bottom; his mind tried to turn it the other way up, but it was impossible.

His mouth twitched and he clenched his teeth to hold in the scream of anger and anguish that churned inside him. He forced himself to tune in again to the low voices of Aileen and Mr Anderson, hers halting and tearful, the consultant replying in his calm and measured way, explaining about MacMillan nurses, the local hospice, making end-of-life plans and getting everything in order.

Unnoticed by him, a nurse dressed in pale blue scrubs and stark white shoes with pink laces had slipped into the room and was now sitting to the side of the consultant's desk, a bundle of leaflets in front of her.

Aileen was holding a leaflet on her lap, spread open so Fin could see a montage of photographs showing a square, modern building set in landscaped gardens, a dining room and bedroom looking like any found in a good, clean hotel. Nurses in lilac uniforms smiled up at him.

The hospice.

They had to pass by it on their way to and from the hospital, but he'd never dreamed he would end up having anything to do with it.

He felt darkness closing in then, and a horrible whining, buzzing noise like a trapped fly filled his ears. He imagined himself falling gracelessly, heavily. Maybe he could pitch forward, crack his skull open on the corner of the desk, so he could stop thinking. What bliss that would be, to not have to think.

But he couldn't do that. It would be selfish. Cowardly.

"How long?" he asked, cutting across something Aileen was saying, his voice sounding as if it had nothing to do with him.

The consultant held Fin's gaze as he said, "It's difficult to say, Fin. Everyone is different."

"Will I see Christmas? New Year?"

Mr Anderson thought for a moment and nodded, bobbing his head quickly down and up again a few times. "Yes. Yes, I think there's a good chance of it. It pays to have something positive to aim for."

So, he might see the New Year in, but the news was still like taking a dagger to the heart, because he wasn't likely to see spring. He had months, just months, and for how many of those would he be well enough to appreciate the extra time?

Aileen, the love of his life, his best friend, his soul mate, would be left alone. He wouldn't be here to watch their son grow up, marry, have a family of his own.

God in heaven, I can't deal with this, he thought.

Aileen clutched at his hand, squeezing his fingers almost to the point of pain. "Fin? Fin! Are you okay?"

A cup of water was placed into his free hand by the nurse. "Sip it slowly," she advised, putting the back of her cool hand to his forehead. "That's right. Now take some deep breaths. Better? Are you sure?"

Fin nodded. He was not going to pass out. How ridiculous that would be. He had been strong for two years; he could manage to be strong for a little while longer. He turned to Aileen and gently wiped her wet cheeks with his thumb. "For us and our wee lad, heh?"

Mr Anderson picked up a pen and wrote something on the top sheet of the file that still lay open on his desk. "I suggest you go home and talk things through. Read those leaflets, they'll tell you everything you need to know. We'll make the arrangements for palliative care, and refer you to the hospice, if that's what you decide. I strongly recommend them, you'll get excellent care and advice, I can guarantee you of that. I'm truly sorry I had to give you such devastating news today."

He closed the file, their signal that all that could be said at this point had been said and a reminder that the consultant had more patients waiting.

Fin and Aileen drove home in silence, Aileen's jaw clenched as she negotiated the traffic, but once through their front door, they simply collapsed into each other's arms and cried. When the tears were spent, albeit temporarily, Aileen made sandwiches and heated up some tinned soup and they sat at the kitchen table, though they were too tired and distressed to eat. Her meal not even half eaten, Aileen pushed the plate away.

"I can't believe it. Why won't they offer more chemo, more radiotherapy, more medication? There's always a chance, isn't there? Fin? Fin! Talk to me!"

Fin examined her face, distressed to see her eyelids swollen and her skin blotchy. Her mouth was turned down at the corners; desperation and despair were all too apparent in her watery, reddened eyes.

Clasping her hand, he said, "They've done all they can, love. Mr Anderson made that very clear and I think we have to accept it. Now, we'll have to call everyone and let them know because we'll need as much support as we can get. God, what am I going to say to Alistair?"

"Do you want him to come back?"

Fin contemplated how much pleasure he would get in spending time with his brother, but contact with him was very much a one-way street. Alistair was constantly on the move, taking work wherever he could find it to fund his next adventure, so Fin relied on his infrequent postcards and phone calls.

"I won't ask him to come. He could be on the other side of the world."

Aileen nodded. She knew what Alistair was like.

Fin said, "We're going to need some help, you know that. I think you should talk to your mum and dad, see if they'll..."

He was stopped mid-sentence by Aileen whipping her hand away from his as her shoulders heaved and she burst into fresh floods of bitter weeping. Then, in one angry gesture she swept all the bowls and plates from the table, sending everything crashing to the floor. Tomato soup spattered the cupboard doors and dripped to the floor.

"Why? Why you? Us? What did we do to deserve this? I can't, I just can't... Oh, Fin, Fin! How can you bear it?"

He moved from his chair and crunched on the broken china to reach her and take her into his arms. But what could he say to comfort her when there was no comfort to be had? She had loved him through everything, even when the first round of chemo had so cruelly affected him. It had taken his hair, eyelashes and eyebrows. Skin that had been firm and healthy had sagged and taken on a sickly yellow hue as he'd not been able to hold any food down. Ribs, knees, hip and cheek bones that had been covered with smooth muscle and flesh stood pointed and sharp, making his once robust and solid body too angular to snuggle up to, even if he'd felt well enough for intimacy.

It had been hell, but he had endured it because he wanted so much to survive, and he'd had reason to believe that the cocktail of drugs would triumph. But the remission had been some kind of practical joke, obviously, for this time the cancer had fought back hard and wormed itself up the spine, heading fast for his brain. Chemo would not beat it this time.

While Aileen fetched a dustpan and brush to start cleaning up, Fin suddenly feeling bone weary, went into the living room and stretched out on the couch, thinking, really thinking, about what meeting the Grim Reaper was going to be like.

Until this moment he'd thought only of standing in defiance before Death, of defeating it and laughing at its retreating back. But everything was different now he knew there would not be a cure, not even another remission. Death would not walk away from him this time. Would letting go be an easy thing, taking that last breath, looking for the last time at the faces of his loved ones? He squeezed his eyes shut and had to swallow hard at the prospect of saying his final goodbyes to Aileen and their wee boy, and of hearing their goodbyes said to him.

As sounds of broken crockery being swept into a dustpan reached him from the kitchen, thoughts of his fast-approaching passing went on swirling in his mind. There would be no more prolonging things with treatment; it wouldn't be worth going through it again even if it was offered, because he knew in his heart that his time had come. He'd accept all the palliative care that could be given and he would stay regularly in the hospice to give Aileen a break; all he asked was that he be allowed to die at home.

He drifted into an exhausted doze then, dreaming of an unfamiliar garden full of people, some of them familiar to him, but there were also some people he didn't know. The dream was peaceful, lulling him deeper into sleep, but suddenly it morphed into something chaotic and incoherent, fast turning into a nightmare.

Then his mother appeared, bringing back the feeling of peace, soothing him with her smiles, her tiny hands cupping his face as she pulled him down so she could kiss him on the forehead. Mairi's lips moved but he could not hear what she was saying, and then he was gently shaken awake by Aileen, telling him she was going to collect Alex from school, and the dream quickly faded.

He looked forward to Alex coming home, filling the house with his energy and excitement as he raced to tell his dad all about his day, to show him a story he'd written or something he'd made. Alex was such a happy boy, he had loads of friends, loved school, loved life, and Fin wanted to howl at the injustice of being forced to leave this Earth while his lad was still so young.

He needed to do something really important for Alex, something truly memorable. He had to plan one spectacular last Christmas for his wee boy.

* * *

"Do you have to go home today, Granny?"

"Yes, we do, my darling boy." Alex snuggled into her lap, giggling as she tickled him. "But we'll be back soon and you can come stay with us in the next holidays. Now then, let's pick up all these toys and pieces of Lego and put them in the box in case Daddy comes down today. You know, don't you, that you need to keep things tidy? And don't be disappointed if there are days that Daddy is too tired to play with you."

Quietened by the reminder that Daddy was very poorly, Alex climbed off her lap and dropped to the floor to gather and put away all his toys. Christmas Day had been the most terrific Christmas Day ever, with snow thick on the ground outside and warmth and light inside, and Mummy and Daddy so cheerful.

Three days had passed since then and the decorations would soon be taken down and put away, but he believed in his young mind that he would always remember every detail. He'd woken early Christmas morning and lay quietly for a few moments, just listening to the house. It hadn't sounded as if anyone else was up yet, but his room was fairly warm, which meant the heating had come on so it wouldn't be long before his mother called him for breakfast. She had been muttering about the boiler playing up, worrying that it would pack up altogether just when there was a blizzard expected in their part of Scotland.

Lying in his cosy bed he'd shivered, but more in excitement and anticipation because his daddy had promised it would be special. He'd pushed his feet all the way down beneath the heavy blankets until he'd felt something heavy with his toes. His Christmas stocking was there, and it was bulging with little presents!

Giggling at the memory of how he'd scoffed all the chocolates and the two satsumas from the stocking before breakfast, Alex revelled in his recollections of that day and Boxing Day and the day after that, and wished again that Granny and Grampy could stay forever.

He finished putting his toys in the toy chest and felt in his trouser pocket for the keyring. Of all the millions of presents he'd opened Christmas morning, this keyring with a blue enamel metal 'A' hanging from it, felt momentous. He was to have his own door key, which meant he was fast becoming a grown-up and Daddy said he would have to be a responsible boy.

He heard Grampy call out that he was bringing the suitcases down, and then his mum appeared at the living room door.

"Oh, good boy Alex, tidying up! You can keep a couple of things out to play with, though." She turned to Alex's granny. "Are you all set? I'm going to miss you so much."

Alex glanced up as the two women hugged, not missing the tear that his mummy quickly wiped away from her cheek.

His granny patted her back. "I wish we didn't have to go, but your dad has to get back to work and we need to secure the house before the blizzard hits. But we'll be back in a flash if you need us, you know that." Alex's granny stepped back from her daughter and gripped her by the upper arms, "Fin is doing well. He's not going anywhere yet a while. Now then, is he coming down today or should we go up to say goodbye? We really should get going."

Alex half wished he could go with them, he loved their place so. The long, untamed garden sloped down to the river and Grampy had a mooring there for his small boat. Alex adored going out on it with him, because he had his own special fishing rod and Granny always sent them off with a smashing packed lunch. But it would be far too cold for boat trips until the spring, and besides, he did understand that he needed to be with Mummy and Daddy right now.

He'd heard what Granny had said, about Daddy not going anywhere, but his other granny, Granny Mairi, had told him that it wouldn't be long and Alex was to be very brave and help Mummy because she was going to be very, very sad.

***

Alex, lying in bed wishing sleep would come, was aware that the days were slipping by and the holidays were coming to an end. Very soon he would be returning to school, and he was both excited and sad at the prospect, for he loved school but he didn't want to be away from his daddy who was so sick.

For about a week following his grandparents' return to their own home, he had been allowed to play with any of his toys as long he kept them over to one area in the living room, away from the couch where Daddy sometimes lay, and if he tidied up immediately when he was asked to. He could go outside and play with his friends, as long as they didn't have colds or coughs and Alex wrapped himself up really well and wore his thick socks and wellies. On the days his daddy had come down, it was always late in the morning, with him taking the stairs very, very slowly. He would stretch out on the couch with a blanket over him, and watch Alex play or listen to him read from one of his many story books. On his really good days he'd managed to play board games like draughts or Monopoly, which Alex loved.

But one day everything had changed. His daddy hadn't come downstairs, and Mummy kept going into the kitchen and closing the door, but Alex could hear her crying and didn't know what to do. At those moments he would rub the smooth enamel 'A' of his keyring, kept always in his pocket; he didn't know why, but it always calmed him.

He'd been allowed to take two or three toys and play in his daddy's room, or sit with him on the bed with a book, as long as he was quiet and left his daddy alone when he was asked to.

Alex was scared, but he always did as he was asked and now, as he lay in his bed with the sound of a fierce gale whipping up outside bedroom window, he was glad when Granny Mairi came and sat by him.

When Granny Mairi had first started visiting him, Alex had learned not to speak out loud to her in case either of his parents heard him. Instead she had taught him how to think his words in a special way, and he heard her replies the same way, in his mind.

"It's telepathy, Alex," she'd explained. *"All you need to do is think about what you want to say to me and I'll hear you just as if we're having a conversation out loud."*

Now, she was telling him not to be afraid and not to worry if he didn't see her for a little while after tonight, because she would be looking after his daddy in heaven. She talked a lot, more than ever before, keeping Alex awake, so he was aware of something happening across the landing in his parents' room, of his mother's weeping. Granny Mairi told him to stay in his bed and listen to her voice, not to pay attention to anything but her. She talked about dying and being alive again in a different way. She told him that his daddy needed to leave his sick body, but that he would be able to visit Alex in spirit, just as she did. Alex would feel very sad, she said, but he had to be a big brave boy.

Thinking his question carefully so Granny Mairi would

hear him, Alex asked, *"Will Daddy feel better when he's left his body?"*

"Oh yes! Much, much better. Remember last summer when you fell over on your new roller skates and hurt yourself? Well, it didn't take long for the pain and bruises to go away, did it? That's because your body is able to get itself better. Your daddy's body can't do that because it doesn't work properly any more."

Alex thought it over. He really had hurt himself that time he'd fallen, scraped and bruised his knees, hands and elbows very badly. His whole body had throbbed and hurt for quite a while, so he imagined that feeling like that for ages and ages would be really horrid.

"Should I tell Mummy all that, Granny Mairi? Would it help her to know that Daddy's body isn't working properly any more so he needs to leave it?'

She sighed softly.

"Oh sweetheart, she knows. Trust me, she knows. But you remember that you shouldn't talk to her about me, don't you, and why?"

Several times in the past she had explained to Alex that some grown-ups didn't always understand about people in spirit so he shouldn't tell anyone about their conversations. When he was older, she said, he'd know how to handle his gift of clairvoyance, but it was best kept secret until then.

She started to sing. Alex didn't understand what the song was about but he loved the soothing tune and the way his granny sang it.

> *"Speed bonnie boat like a bird on the wing*
> *Onward the sailors cry.*
> *Carry the lad that's born to be king*

*Over the sea to Skye.
Loud the winds howl, loud the waves roar,
Thunderclaps rend the air . . ."*

The wind was now howling outside, but it didn't scare him because Granny Mairi made him feel so loved, so safe. He whispered that he didn't want her to go away.

"I know, Alex, but your daddy needs me more than you do right now, and it'll only be for a wee while, I promise. I need you to be brave for your mummy. Will you promise me you'll be a good boy and look after her?"

Singing the second verse, she rose from his bedside and started to fade as she floated away from him. Alex had to fight to stop his bottom lip wobbling. Her last words before she faded completely were nothing more than a whisper and Alex could no longer keep his tired eyes from closing.

When he awoke the room was freezing cold. The window sills outside were covered with deep drifts of snow and his breath made little vapour clouds in front of his face. It was still dark, so either it was still very, very early in the morning and the heating hadn't yet come on, or the boiler had finally stopped working as his mummy had feared it would.

Alex wanted to snuggle down into the warm blankets and stay there, but he slowly became aware of a change in the atmosphere of his room and of a faint misty glow forming like a cloud at the bottom of his bed.

Alex blinked to see Granny Mairi and Grampy Donald standing behind his daddy, the three of them surrounded by the mist. His daddy smiled at him with a mixture of sadness and pure joy.

"I'm free, Alex. It's wonderful."

Chapter 3
FLORA
Manchester, 2009

Flora kept watch while her mummy prised away one of the planks that had been nailed across a window. The two of them were at the back of the house, well-hidden in the shadows, at the end of an abandoned terrace, but Rachel warned Flora there might be a security guard on patrol.

Rachel swore under her breath as a fingernail broke, but once she'd got her fingers firmly curled behind the end of the plank she was able to yank it free. The next ones were much easier and soon she'd made enough of a gap for them to climb through, saying a soft and relieved "Hallelujah!" when she found there was no glass in the old wooden frame. She hoisted Flora up onto the rotting wooden sill and she nimbly jumped down into what had once been a small kitchen. Dust puffed up around her feet, and her nose wrinkled against the musty smell.

Switching on her precious torch, which she could tell would soon need new batteries, Flora swung the beam around to get her bearings. Pipes below the window she had just climbed through showed that the sink had once been there; the doors of the floor-standing kitchen units hung crookedly from their hinges; dust and mouse droppings covered every surface. There was only one door to the room, directly opposite where she'd jumped in.

Flora stood back as the black plastic dustbin bags holding their possessions were dropped in, then Rachel heaved herself through the window and landed lightly in front of her.

The torch beam flickered. "Mum, I need new batteries."

"Oh, you and your torch!" said Rachel, teasing laughter in her voice. "You know we haven't got any; I'll see what I can do tomorrow." She bent down and kissed the tip of Flora's nose. "Haven't I always promised I wouldn't leave you in the dark? I'll get some for you when I can, I promise."

Flora, wanting to conserve whatever was left of her torch's power, put it back in the pocket of her anorak. She took the two bin bags her mother handed her and followed her into the hallway. Beneath the fine layer of dust she could see that its floor tiles were cracked and stained, and there were dark stains on the walls in many places too. Rachel tried to open the first door but it jammed against something behind it and no matter how hard she pushed she couldn't get enough clearance to get inside. The door on the other side swung open unimpeded, but the room was pitch-dark because of its boarded-up window.

"Give me the torch."

Flora reluctantly handed it over, but when Rachel clicked it on the beam flickered for just a moment before dimming and disappearing altogether. She shook it but that didn't help.

"Damn, it's too dark in here and we certainly can't sleep in the kitchen. Never mind, we'll have to try upstairs."

She quickly closed the door again and Flora could see that she was making a funny face at her in the gloom.

"Come on, munchkin. We've at least an hour before it

gets fully dark, so we'll get settled before then. It's been quite a day and we need to sleep, then I'll sort everything all out in the morning, okay?"

She led the way up the stairs, testing each step carefully before putting her full weight on it. Flora knew her mother preferred that they sleep downstairs to give them an easier escape route should they need it, but there was no way they could stay in the pitch dark of that room without first seeing what was in it, nor would they be able to sleep in the mouse-infested kitchen with a gaping window.

The uncarpeted stairs creaked beneath their feet, but at least the last of the daylight still filtered through planks haphazardly nailed on the inside of the window at the top of the staircase, giving them enough light to see by. There were two bedrooms upstairs, one tiny and filled with broken furniture, the other a good size and empty except for a mattress and a dead pigeon lying in its own droppings.

"Hey, look at that!" said Rachel, pointing to the mattress. "What luck!" She dumped the bags she was carrying, beckoning Flora to do the same. "It may not be cosy but at least it's dry. Here, help me tip this up and I'll brush it off. It'll be fine if we lay our clothes on top of it." She paused, seeing the doubt on Flora's face. "I know this is horrid, munchkin, but it's getting dark, it feels like rain is coming, so we'll just have to make the best of it. We'll have all day tomorrow to find somewhere better."

Wordlessly, Flora helped to clear the mattress of dust, dirt and droppings, and Rachel tipped one of the bags of clothes onto it and spread them out. Flora rolled up two sweaters for them to use as pillows. She was so tired she would have lain in the dust on the floor if she'd had to, but she was grateful for the softness of the mattress, if not for the nasty smell that came from it.

They ate some chocolate biscuits and an apple each, then, exhausted by the bewildering day she'd just had, Flora curled herself into the warmth of Rachel's back and closed her eyes. She expected to fall instantly into a deep sleep, as her mummy did, but was dismayed to find herself wide awake and staring into the blackness.

She curled her arm around her mother's waist, snuggling closer, wondering how they had ended up here, forced to spend a night in such a horrid place. How had she and her mother ended up breaking into an abandoned house for shelter? They'd lived in a nice flat once, and Flora had gone to the local primary school, well-fed and in smart, clean clothes. Then, as far as she'd understood it, her mum had lost her job, been unable to pay the rent, and had been thrown out by the horrible landlord. It might also have had something to do with her mum's boyfriend who came and went and smoked something that made him behave a bit odd.

Anyway, following the eviction the boyfriend was never seen again and they'd stayed with friends for a little while, both of them sleeping on the big sofa in the front room. Flora had liked the friends, and loved their fluffy, purring grey cat that liked to curl up in her lap, but they'd all too soon moved on from there because, Rachel explained, they mustn't ever impose on friends for longer than a week. Flora hadn't understood that, for if they were friends, surely they wouldn't mind how long they stayed? She and her mother were scrupulously tidy, and Flora was careful not to make any noise or get in anyone's way.

From there they had moved to a tiny basement room of a three-storey house that seemed to Flora to be home to about two dozen people, but then, in the dead of night, her mum had ordered her to help pack up their few possessions and they had crept away once Rachel had gone round like a burglar searching in drawers, pockets and under sofa cushions for any cash.

Flora had been frightened in case they'd been caught, but Rachel had said, "They're all stoned, don't worry about it." Flora worried that her mother had hit them all with a stone.

For a time after that it seemed to Flora that they never spent more than a night or two on a sofa or blow-up mattress on the floor, her mum telling her to wait in another room while men came to chat to her in private. She always seemed unhappy after the men had been, but they must have enjoyed talking to her because they always gave her some money. Some of the men offered a lot more money to talk with Flora, but this was one thing Rachel would not allow, turning into a spitting, raging hellcat as she shoved them out, barricaded the door and quickly moved her and Flora on again.

For this Flora was grateful, for sometimes she heard things that frightened her and she didn't like the men at all. She quickly learned to be well out of sight before they saw her and stay hidden until they had gone.

School became a distant memory. Flora was dressed every day in grey trousers and baggy sweaters and she had cried when her hair had been cropped really short so she looked like a boy. Rachel had cried too, as she cut it with a large pair of scissors, muttering that she could not risk Flora looking like a pretty little girl when there were so many bad men around.

Her mum had been pretty once. Flora remembered when her thick, reddish-blond hair, the same texture and colour as her own, flowing in shining waves to just below her mother's shoulders. Her eyes were huge, blue or deep green depending on what she was wearing or what mood she was in, and long-lashed. There was a smattering of freckles across her neat nose, and she had small, even, white teeth. When she smiled her whole face lit up. Flora remembered a time when they had cuddled up together and she'd felt the cushioning of well-fed flesh and muscle.

Rachel did not look or feel like that now, and she rarely smiled. Her hair, though still long, had streaks of grey in it and was often dull and greasy at the roots. She had become skinny and her eyes, once so soft and happy, had turned hard, the skin around them sometimes black and blue with bruises that she explained away by saying she was tired.

One day she had disappeared for hours, wearing her long coat, ordering Flora not to move from the room. When she came back, she looked quite plump until she'd shrugged off the coat. Flora had gasped as she removed layer after layer of clothes. She'd piled them on the single bed they were sharing, then sat down on the floor and started to remove the price labels by biting through the plastic tags with the good teeth she still had on the left side of her mouth.

When Flora turned nine years old, Rachel took her into a supermarket and told her to choose a birthday cake from the many on display on the shelves. Flora had looked up at her, wide-eyed with fear, but her mum had dipped her hand into her jacket pocket and brought out some money. She held the coins in her open palm so Flora could see and understand that the cake would be paid for. She'd chosen the smallest one, vanilla sponge with strawberry jam in the middle, covered in pink frosting, with a simple 'Happy Birthday' written in white curly script across the top. They'd eaten the whole lot between them in one go.

At that time they were living with a huge, red-faced man everyone called Hemp, and although Flora didn't like him, she was glad to have her own clean bed to sleep in and a bathroom with hot running water to wash in.

Her mother started to look better too, the hollows in her face filled out and her smile flashed more often, so Flora dared to hope that their fortunes had turned around and this would be her permanent home. She was allowed to be a girl again, she even had a couple of dresses and nice shoes, and was allowed to let her hair grow, though it seemed to take a very long time.

There was talk of school, which excited her so much, but she never got to go. Hemp had begun to look too closely at her, his eyes following her every move with an expression that made her increasingly nervous, so this morning, once again, they had fled in the very early hours, taking what money her mother could find but leaving behind some of their best clothes and Flora's much-loved pair of pink, fluffy slippers. She so loved pink, probably because of all the time she'd been forced to wear boys clothing in boring navy blue, brown and dark green.

They'd walked a long time, then Rachel had put them onto a bus, paying for tickets that would take them to the bus station. From there they had walked and walked, lugging all the possessions her mother had managed to stuff into four large bin liners, until they turned up a street that was lined on both sides by boarded up terraced houses. Graffiti had been sprayed on every wall and across all the 'keep out' signs nailed to the doors, but they'd broken into the last house on the left, its two bay windows solidly boarded up so their only option was to go round the back and get in through the kitchen window. And here they were, holed up in a derelict house on a mattress that was filled with who knew what kinds of creepy-crawlies.

Flora must have drifted off to sleep at last, for suddenly she was being shaken awake. She sat up, teeth chattering because of a chilly and damp draught coming in through a hole in the window pane. Heavy rain drummed against the window and the roof. Rachel handed her a biscuit and what was left of their bottle of water, whispering that she was going out to find them something to eat.

"There's no point in us both getting soaked so you stay here, Flora. You mustn't go anywhere, understand me? I'm not sure how far it is to the nearest shop, but I promise I'll be as quick as I can. We'll have breakfast, whatever I can get, and then we'll move on as soon as the rain stops and find somewhere better to stay tonight."

She pinched Flora's chin and kissed the tip of her nose, then quietly left the room.

Flora listened to her mother's footsteps on the stairs until they faded, then snuggled back down under the pile of clothes and, despite the chill of the room and the gnawing hunger in her tummy, was soon asleep again.

When she next woke up it was because it was raining even harder and there was pressure on her bladder she couldn't ignore. Was she not meant to leave this room at all, which would mean going to the toilet right here, or would it be all right if she went to the bathroom? Where was the bathroom? She didn't remember seeing one. Some of the houses they'd stayed in had bathrooms downstairs at the back, but she was sure there'd been no other doors leading from the kitchen besides the one to the hallway.

She didn't know how long she lay there in indecision, in that damp space, mice droppings all around, trying to keep her mind from thinking how desperate she was to pee. She wasn't helped by the sound of the incessant rain, so she rose, wincing as she unfolded herself from the mattress because her limbs had become painfully stiff. Shivering, she quickly pulled on another sweater under her anorak and crept out of the room.

There was a closed door next to the smaller bedroom so she peeked inside and was relieved to see a toilet. The room was hardly wider than her outstretched arms, the toilet had no seat and the water in it was a dark, murky brown with an oily film on top. On the floor was a roll of toilet paper, damp and flecked with grey. Thick cobwebs swayed above her head, but she didn't care, her need was too great now to bother about spiders, so great in fact that she almost didn't get her pink jeans unzipped and pulled down in time.

Once relieved, she looked for the flush handle, but the cistern was very high up on the wall and the pull chain out of reach, even if she stood on tiptoe. She contemplated standing on the toilet bowl, but could imagine slipping and her foot going into that horrid brown water that she'd just added to.

She scurried back to the bedroom to wait. After a while, when too much time seemed to pass, she crept to the window and peered out, careful not to show too much of herself. Her lip curled as she noticed how close her foot was to the dead, decomposing pigeon beneath the window sill, its scaly clawed feet pointing to the ceiling.

The room was at the front of the house, so the window looked out onto the deserted street and the blank faces of the boarded-up houses opposite. There were no cars, no people, in fact no movement at all that she could see. Not having a watch she had no idea what time it was, but it felt as if her mother had been gone a very, very long time. Maybe the shops were miles away? She'd be soaked through and they'd not brought any towels away from Hemp's place.

More time passed. She ate the last two biscuits in the packet, now slightly stale, and folded up the clothes they'd used as their sheets, placing them carefully in the bin bags. Still Rachel didn't come and she was getting scared. Really scared.

There was a noise downstairs, a scraping sound, and her spirits rose in anticipation of her mother's return and something good to eat. But there was no bright voice calling her to come up, so Flora crept out of the bedroom and peered down into the narrow, gloomy hall. She listened hard but her ears caught no more sounds. Maybe her mother had gone into the kitchen, though she couldn't think why as she'd seen nothing useful in there yesterday.

The banister rail wobbled as she touched it, so she went down each step carefully, keeping herself close to the wall. From the hallway she could only see a glimpse of the kitchen, but the living room door was wide open, and unlike the blackness of the day before, there was light within. Feeling confident that her mum was in there, having bought candles and other supplies, and making everything as nice as it could be before she called Flora down to join her, she skipped down the last few stairs, clearing the bottom two steps with one jump.

Her mother was not there, but Flora didn't worry about it, just looked with delight at the things in front of her, glad of the single candle that lit the room. There was a sleeping bag rolled up and secured with string on the hearth of the fireplace, a large canvas satchel leaning against it. In front of the hearth was a cooker ring connected to a small, round, bright blue gas bottle, a carton of milk and pizza box. Why hadn't she come up straight away to check on Flora? And to bring her down to show her what she'd brought?

Flora darted forward to lift the lid on the box, disappointed to find that there was only a quarter slice of pizza left in it. Had her mother eaten the rest of it and left just that little bit for her? Her stomach grumbled, a mixture of real hunger, annoyance and nagging fear; where had her mummy gone?

"Mum?" she called, her voice wavering. She cleared her throat and tried again. "Mummy! Where are you? I'm scared!"

Flora waited, hardly daring to breathe. She could only think that Rachel was fetching in more things and she'd just have to wait.

She spotted the pile of yellowing newspapers and a little stack of wood to the right of the fireplace; how lovely it would be to have a fire to drive away the dampness of this room. She gazed hungrily at the pizza, then snatched up the slice and ate it quickly, stuffing it all in her mouth at once so it filled both her cheeks. It was cold and soggy and didn't taste very nice, but she used her fingers to wipe the congealed remnants of sauce and a few strands of hard cheese from the box. She tore open the carton of milk and drank deep; it was deliciously cold and refreshing.

Now she decided to investigate the dark green canvas bag, wondering where her mum had got it from and hoping there would be batteries for her torch inside. When she had undone the two buckled straps, she pulled out its contents and set them on the floor: battered tin cup; box of matches; pouch of strong-smelling tobacco; flat packet of cigarette papers, of the kind she had seen often in the various places they'd stayed; multi-bladed penknife with a scratched, red handle that had a white cross on it; plastic disposable razor with black whiskers caught between the twin blades; a small, locked, square tin that was heavy and rattled when she shook it; a metal ring with lots of small keys on it; a bottle half full of purple liquid.

At the bottom of the bag she found several items of men's clothing, all filthy and greasy to the touch. Eyeing these things left her in no doubt that her mum had stolen the bag from someone. She swallowed hard.

There was that scraping noise again, and she could tell someone was in the kitchen. She froze at the sound of heavy footsteps tramping along the hall, for she knew they couldn't belong to her cat-footed mother. They stopped outside the half-closed door and Flora felt her mouth go dry.

What should she do? Announce herself straight away and apologise that she had touched his things, or hide until she could see what type of person he was? Where, oh where was her mum? What if she had stolen these things and the owner had followed her here to get them back, or Hemp had managed to trace them and had hurt her before coming for Flora?

Frantically, she checked round the room, a perfect square except for the bay window, no nooks or crannies, no cupboards. No way could she climb into the fireplace and crawl up inside the chimney. No way could she push her way out of the boarded-up window. There really was nowhere for her to hide, no way out but past whoever was standing in the hall, someone she could hear breathing heavily on the other side of the door.

Deciding her only hope was to make a run for it, she crept to the door, keeping her head down, ready to whip the door open and barge past whoever was waiting out there, scared witless that even if she got past that obstacle, she might be caught before she made it to the kitchen and out of the window.

The candle went out.

With a deep breath she made her move, and careered full pelt into the bulk of a man that seemed like a giant to her, whose foul body odour almost made her gag. Her head ramming into his stomach forced the breath from his lungs with a whooshing, hissing sound, but he didn't fall or stagger away from her and all she had time to register, as he grabbed her and pushed her violently away from him was the rough texture of his clothes, his long black hair and the expression on his dirty, horribly scarred and pitted face.

Chapter 4
WALTER AND VERITY
Wiltshire, 2013

Yawning until her jaw hurt, Kallie wondered what had been the cause of last night's nightmare that had her waking in a sweat in the early hours, fighting the duvet that was wrapped tightly round her legs.

She cast a quick glance at her grandmother sitting so serenely in the passenger seat, humming quietly to the music. It wasn't her choice, she was so tired she'd prefer something modern, loud and lively that she could sing along to, but classical music calmed Verity so she always had a couple of CDs in the car for when she was a passenger.

Verity was very frail these days, and Kallie worried for her as her grandfather's death seemed imminent. How would she cope when her soul mate was gone? Kallie shuddered at what was to come and her stomach fluttered with butterflies. Since she'd been little, she coloured her imaginary butterflies in different shades: red for excitement, yellow for nervous tension, muddy brown for sadness, bright blue for joy. Today's butterflies were dark grey and black. Or maybe they weren't butterflies, but moths or miniature bats. She shuddered at the unwelcome image of bats with their huge ears and leathery wings and forced herself to concentrate on the country roads they were travelling along.

At last they arrived at their destination and she swung the car between the ivy-covered stone gateposts of Rainstones House and headed for the car park. It appeared to be full already, but just as Verity was starting to fret—as she fretted about every little thing these days—that they might not find anywhere to park, someone walking by tapped on the window and told Kallie that if she drove all the way past the dementia care wing she'd find a space at the far end.

It turned out to be a tricky one between a white minivan and a low stone wall, but Kallie manoeuvred her small car into it with ease. Careful not to clip the wall as she opened the door she squeezed out and walked round to help her grandmother get out. She gave her the walking stick, then took her other arm, and they walked slowly back to the hospice wing of the complex, Kallie cross with herself for not thinking to drop Verity off at Reception before parking.

Once inside, Verity insisted she was all right to go on ahead on her own and Kallie, taking that to mean that her gran wanted some time alone with Walter, took her time writing their names and the car registration into the visitor's book before following her.

By the time she entered the corridor Verity was out of sight, so she must have marched along at a surprisingly fast pace, wanting only to get to her husband's bedside as quickly as possible. Kallie slowed her own pace right down, intending to give her grandparents a good ten minutes alone together.

At his request and because of the good fortune of there being a bed available, Walter had been brought in four days earlier because he was convinced he didn't have much longer. Verity had resisted letting him go, she so wanted him to spend his last days at home, but from the start of his illness Walter had demanded from her a promise that she grant him his wish to die in this beautiful place. He'd made sure Kallie understood what he wanted, too, asking her to please make sure his wishes were carried out because it would be best for all of them, even if Verity couldn't see it yet.

"I'll likely be in nappies and needing God knows what kind of care by then and I don't want my Verity nursing me through that," he'd growled to Kallie when Verity had left the room to take a phone call, his eyebrows low over his fierce gaze. "And I certainly don't want you nursing me either, washing and changing me, though I know you'd do it with good heart and without a murmur of complaint."

Verity had come back in then and he'd said, "I'm not dying in our bed, woman! I want you to be able to sleep there and remember me fondly when I'm gone. Besides, have you given any consideration to how they'd get a stretcher up and down our stairs?" He'd snorted at the thought. "I shall die peacefully and with dignity in the hospice, I know it and you know it, so there are to be no arguments when the time comes."

And there had been no arguments when the time came, for Verity, worn out despite all the extra help Kallie had arranged, had capitulated with her usual quiet grace when Walter asked her to make arrangements for his immediate admission, and Kallie had felt it right to back him up.

The tiny old cottage the three of them had shared since Kallie's birth, with its bathroom downstairs beyond the kitchen and steep and narrow stairs up to the bedroom, was hardly suitable for caring for someone as sick as Walter.

At the beginning of his illness he'd spent a day each week

in the Day Patient Unit to give Verity a break, a day which had her worrying rather than relaxing, but he had enjoyed it very much, and really, he'd been right that going to the hospice as an inpatient was the only sensible option.

Kallie had never seen the Day Patient Unit, which her grandfather referred to as 'the jolly old DPU', because she was always working, but Walter told her how he enjoyed spending time there because everyone was just lovely.

Kallie's throat tightened as she wondered how much longer her precious grandfather had. Since his arrival by special ambulance he'd gone downhill fast, and the last two days he'd only been conscious for short periods of time. It had been heart-breaking watching Verity grasp his hands, kiss his face, all the while telling him it was okay for him to go. But he was still here, still fighting to have a little more time with his beloved wife and granddaughter.

Still dragging her feet, Kallie paused half way along the passageway, where another corridor led off to the right, leading to the therapy rooms, the DPU and the chapel. She could smell the sweet perfumes of aromatherapy oils, so familiar to her, and longed to see inside the rooms and meet the therapists. She knew that anyone in the hospice could ask for treatments both practical, such as manicure and pedicure, and holistic, including aromatherapy, reflexology and acupuncture. Maybe she could offer her services? How wonderful that would be. She thought she could work it so she had two half days a week here, even one full day, and still keep all her clients happy at the salon, where she worked with another beautician and two hair stylists.

The sweet smells disappeared immediately as she pushed open the door into the Inpatient Unit, which always smelled different to anywhere else in the hospice wing. It wasn't unpleasant, just a mixture of odours that marked the place as a medical area.

The beautifully decorated single rooms were on one side of the modern, purpose-built wing that had been added to the old stone building about a decade before. Each had a hospital bed, wall-mounted television, radio and DVD player, small ensuite bathroom, and sliding glass doors that opened out onto a private patio. Here, if the weather was warm and dry, patients and their visitors could sit and have their meals, read books of their own or borrowed from the many donated to the library, or simply gaze at the spectacular, beautifully landscaped grounds against their backdrop of rolling Wiltshire hills.

The door to her grandfather's room opened as she approached and a young nurse came out, carrying a shallow metal bowl covered with a cloth.

"Hello, Kallie," she whispered. "Your grandad's asleep at the moment, but he might wake up soon. He had a peaceful night."

Kallie could only nod as her throat was so tight now she was unable to force any words out. Showing complete understanding, the nurse gave her a sympathetic smile and told Kallie to come and find her if anything was needed during her visit.

She crept into the room and kissed Walter before carrying on outside so Verity could be alone with him but call her back in if she needed to. Turning a patio chair so she could see into the room as well as into the garden she sat with her elbow on the little metal table and gazed towards the water sculpture, the symbol of Rainstones House Hospice & Dementia Care since its installation in the early 1980s.

It was a slender tower of unusually shaped quartz stones

hung with small copper bells. The stones glistened and sparkled in the water that flowed over them from the top of a pipe running through its centre. The falling water caused the bells to knock against the quartz, making the most beautiful sound. She knew from the literature Verity had been given when they'd first investigated the place that the name Rainstones was a bit of a mystery, but the sculpture had been commissioned and donated by the grateful relative of a patient. She thought she might stroll over there before leaving today, just to see it up close and hear its music more clearly than she could from where she was sitting.

Being the first room nearest the entrance to the unit, her grandfather's terrace was sheltered by the golden stone wall of the older part of the building that housed the therapy rooms and other areas of the hospice, and it was exceptionally warm today. She tipped her face up to the sun, closing her eyes tight until the colour behind her eyelids flared and glowed deep orange and vibrant red.

She was glad she'd been able to clear her diary to have these few days off, because she didn't think she'd be able to work competently knowing her grandmother was sitting alone in vigil by Walter's bedside, hour after hour, until Kallie could get back here again.

Someone coughed from the patio next door, screened from Kallie by a low wall and trellis that dripped with clematis. Kallie opened her eyes and observed a group of gardeners arriving to start work on the large ornamental flower beds. They were all volunteers, she knew, and thought what a wonderful job that would be.

Hearing the bedroom door open she swung her head to see who had arrived. It was Bronwyn, the lovely senior nurse who'd been looking after them all from the day Walter had been referred by his doctor for hospice care. Kallie had quickly come to admire her steady manner and straightforward approach to her job. Bronwyn said a few words to Verity and then came outside.

"I'm just about to finish my shift, but I like to check on all my patients before I leave. How are you, Kallie?"

If that question were asked anywhere else and by anyone else she would reply with the usual, 'Fine, thanks. How are you?' But here they genuinely wanted to know, and Bronwyn's open gaze and soft Welsh lilt made you want to open up to her with honesty, so her reply was, "Shit-scared."

It sounded shocking spoken within earshot of Verity, who did not approve of even the mildest bad language no matter what the circumstance. Bronwyn hugged her, a deeply personal gesture Kallie would never have expected from her, and she had to bite her lip hard to keep the ever-present tears at bay.

"Your grandfather is where he wants to be, and it's the best possible place. You know that, don't you? He's in no pain and we'll take very good care of him in the time he has left." Bronwyn glanced back at Verity. "Your grandmother is an amazing lady, isn't she?"

Kallie nodded and swallowed hard so she could speak.

"She really is. She's worn out with worry, but, you know, she always wants to look beautiful for him. She chooses her outfit the night before we come, making sure it's pressed and her shoes are polished, and she sits at her dressing table to do her hair and make-up while I dash about like a headless chicken. I'm worried that she's become so frail, but she's always calm, far more stoic than I am, yet her loss will be far greater. I hear her telling him it's okay for him to go, that she'll be fine because she knows it won't be long before she joins him, and it breaks my heart." A sob caught in Kallie's throat on the last word.

Bronwyn patted her arm and smiled. "It's her way of reassuring him. I've seen it all since I've worked here. Some, like Verity, can let go of their loved ones calmly and with dignity, others just need to rant and rave at their going. We're all different, and of course it depends on age; far harder to let go of someone young. But if you're worried about your gran's health we can check her over." She quickly checked her watch. "I really must go, or my daughter will be very cross with me. I'm on call, though, and I'll come straight back if I'm needed. Stay strong, Kallie. It's all you can do."

Kallie managed a small smile, but by telling her she was on call, Bronwyn was letting her know that she expected Walter to die very, very soon. The thought made her stomach churn anew.

Verity was coping admirably now, at least outwardly, but did she mean it when she said she'd soon be joining Walter? They had been together since Verity was sixteen, Walter a couple of years older, but now the time they had left was ticking away hour by hour, minute by minute, to a matter of—what? A couple more days? Maybe only a handful of hours? The bats in her stomach chittered and stirred their leathery wings at her troubled thoughts that it could be that very day.

Moments after Bronwyn had gone, leaving the room after a quick check on Walter and a quiet word to Verity, Kallie crept back into the room and leaned back against the wall, taking in the scene of the still figure lying on the bed, the beautiful lady sitting so serenely beside it.

Her grandfather had lost so much weight he barely made a mound under the sheet and thin blanket that covered him. But then, so had Verity. Kallie saw for the first time how her clothes hung off her shoulders, even her shoes seemed a size too big. She saw movement in the bed as Walter flexed his legs, then his eyelids flickered and opened, his gaze searching for and locking on to Verity.

"Hello, sweetheart," he whispered, and Kallie had to swallow hard at how much she was moved by all the love contained in those two simple words.

Her grandmother's face was luminous as she smiled at Walter, and Kallie could only wish that one day she would find a love like theirs.

"I've been having the most wonderful dreams," Walter whispered. "A garden, oh the most beautiful garden you've ever seen. It's full of people, ordinary people just like me, and I see my mum and dad, my brother. But there are also these ..." He stopped and shrugged his thin shoulders. "Oh, I don't know what they are or how to describe them. Maybe they're angels!"

He grinned at Verity and Kallie, his face boyish for a moment.

"There's a bright light waiting for me, just like you read about, and I'm not at all afraid. Truly, I'm not afraid, my love. But they're not taking me yet."

He noticed Kallie then, and beckoned her over.

Kallie, marvelling both at the length of her grandfather's speech and at what he was saying, crept up to the bed and bent down to kiss the whiskery, paper-dry cheek. She noticed that his lips were dry and cracked, so she moistened a cotton pad in water, always kept handy on the bedside table, and tenderly dabbed the mouth of the elderly man she loved so, so much.

"Shall I massage your feet for you, Grandad? I've brought some mint-scented lotion just for you, I know you'll love the smell."

"Maybe in a little while, darling." His voice was weak and raspy. "Right now there's something else I'd like very much."

Kallie smiled down at him, wondering what it could be.

"I'd love a cup of tea!"

Her grandmother reached for her stick and started to rise, saying she would go and find someone to make it so Kallie could sit and have a chat with her grandad, but Walter stopped her with a surprisingly strong gesture.

"Kallie will make it, won't you, lass? Make a proper pot, my darling, no dunking teabags in mugs!"

"Of course, Grandad!" She couldn't keep the happy surprise out of her voice.

All he'd wanted these past couple of days was a little lemonade mixed with tepid water. Perhaps this was a good sign. Hadn't he just said that he wasn't going yet?

"I'll see to it straightaway." Kallie headed for the door, but was called back by that thin, reedy voice.

"I love you, Kallie, you're a special girl."

She blew him a kiss. "I love you too, with all my heart. I'll be back in two minutes."

Kallie hurried to the small kitchen provided for visitors and deciding to make a bit of an occasion of it as her grandad clearly wanted, she located a small milk jug, three cups with matching saucers, a stainless-steel strainer, and a china teapot that she warmed through before making the tea with leaves, not bags. She found a freshly laundered white cloth with which to cover the tray, and a small box of shortbread. Taking just three biscuits, she lifted the tray and headed back.

She entered the room backwards, pushing the door open with her hip, swinging away from the bed as she came in so she could place the laden tray down on top of the chest of drawers. Quickly, she set the cups on saucers, added milk and poured tea through the strainer, wondering if her grandfather would be able to manage to keep the delicate cup in his grip.

"Tea for three, just as you ordered!" she sang. "It's Assam. Shortbread biscuits too. Shame we can't all sit out on the patio, it's such a lovely day and the garden looks beautiful, but we'll have our own little tea party right here."

She turned back to the bed, a cup and saucer in each hand. It took her a full two seconds to realise that her gran was crying, crying so quietly Kallie hadn't heard her while her back was turned, and another second to comprehend that her grandfather had gone. Really gone.

Forcing herself to place the cups back on the tray rather than just let them tumble from her numbed hands and smash on the floor, she understood that he had sent her away so he could be alone with his Verity as he'd taken his last breath.

* * *

Feeling as if she were in some kind of hideous time loop, Kallie once again moved amongst the same mourners who had come to Walter's funeral just three months before. The cottage being far too small for so many people she had hired the parish hall for both funerals, made the same buffet refreshments, gone through the same motions the whole day through, and now her beloved grandparents were resting side by side in the graveyard just over the wall that divided the church and its grounds from the cottage garden.

Three months, that's all it had taken for Verity to achieve her aim of joining her husband. With the benefit of hindsight, Kallie believed that her gran, already frail, had held on just to see that Walter's funeral was conducted the way she wanted, with utmost dignity, and then she had simply forced her body by sheer willpower to shut down.

All of Kallie's pleading for Verity not to leave her had done no good, and once Verity had had her say, Kallie realised she had no choice but to let her grandmother go to where she truly wanted to be.

"Kallie," Verity had said, taking Kallie's hands in hers with surprising strength. "I am old. I want to be with my Walter. I've kept it from you for some time, but there is something wrong with me. I'm not in pain, I assure you, so I ask you, beg you, not to let the doctor anywhere near me. Just let me go quietly, my dear. You have your whole life ahead of you and one day soon you'll meet your own soulmate and if I'm still here you'll be torn between setting up home with him, as you should, and looking after me. I don't want that for you, my darling girl, I want for you and me both to be free."

Verity refused to have the same helpers who had cared for Walter to come back and look after her, asking only that Kallie help her dress and get downstairs and leave her a little lunch before she went to work. Not wanting to leave her gran all day, Kallie arranged her appointments at the salon so she could get back in the middle of the day, and she made sure she was always home on time in the evenings.

For a while it seemed as if Verity was perking up, for she talked about Walter as if he was with her all the time. *Maybe he was*, Kallie thought, but even if he was just a figment of the imagination it made Gran happy, so she would laugh and ask what Walter had to say for himself.

The morning Verity died, they'd had breakfast together as usual, Verity eating very little. Kallie had settled her in the living room with a blanket over her legs, a flask of tea and the television remote control close to hand, though Verity preferred to listen to the radio. She had made two rounds of sandwiches and put them on a plate, covered, with two pots of fruit yogurt on the kitchen table, ready for her and Verity to have for their lunch. She'd be able to get home for no more than half an hour, she'd said as she was leaving.

She'd come home at half past twelve to find Verity dead and cold in the chair, looking as if she hadn't moved from the moment Kallie had helped her sit there. Maybe she hadn't. Kallie had been gone just a few hours, her gran could have drawn her last breath at any time in those hours.

"People are leaving now, Kallie."

Blinking, Kallie came out of her abstraction to notice that the crowd of black-clad mourners were gathering their things and preparing to go home. She moved quickly to the door to stand by her mother to say thank you and goodbye, wanting now for them all to be gone so she could tidy up and go back to the cottage.

Once the hall was empty of people, she went round the tables scraping the remnants of sandwiches, quiches and cakes, into the middle of the paper table cloths, then balling the cloths up ready to take outside to the large bin. Her friends and a couple of neighbours offered to help, but Kallie thanked them and ordered them away, saying she and her mother would get it all done between them

She collected and boxed all the plates, cups and glasses that she'd hired along with the hall so she could take it all home to wash before returning it; there was no sign of Celia. The hall was only a short distance from the cottage, but Kallie had to cart out and load the heavy boxes into her car and drive round.

It wasn't until she had carried in the last box that her mother appeared, her face tear-stained and blotchy, her nose bright pink, making her look plainer than ever. Kallie had no idea where she'd been, and was further irritated when Celia simply leaned against the fridge with her arms crossed watching her unpack the boxes and load the dishwasher instead of offering any assistance.

She didn't speak until Kallie picked up a couple of wine glasses, and then she said, "I trust you're going to wash those by hand. The dishwasher will ruin them."

Kallie's brewing temper blew then, and she berated Celia for not contributing anything to the day, as she hadn't for Walter's funeral, her tirade ending in tears as she thought of how horrified Verity would be if she'd been there to witness this anger and frustration.

Not moving from her place against the fridge, Celia said, "I don't think you know how hard it was for me to learn that Dad had died before I'd had a chance to say goodbye, and then to lose Mum so soon afterwards, with no warning. I should have been around more."

"Yes, you should! Have you given any thought to how it's been for me? Gran called you the day Grandad went into the hospice, but you didn't come straight away, did you? And then you say you were overcome with grief when I called to tell you Gran had died, but you hadn't been to visit her for over a week to see how she was coping. She was grieving, I was grieving, so how come this is all about you? I came home from work to find her dead, have you thought what that was like for me? I left her alone for just a couple of hours. When I found her it was as if she hadn't moved from her chair from the time I left for work in the morning and came back to give her some lunch. I've had to deal with everything, Mum, with no help from you! I had to make all the arrangements twice over, and now you're here crying that you weren't around much! Well that choice was yours, wasn't it? It was always yours."

She stood rigid in front of Celia, her hands in fists at her sides. Both of them were shocked by her outburst, Kallie herself having no idea how or why their mutual grief had degenerated into such a flare up. But wasn't it always the way with them? They were just toxic together.

Without a word her mother walked away, leaving Kallie to get on with washing the glasses in hot, soapy water. When Celia came back she was carrying her overnight bag.

"It's too late for me to drive all the way to Cambridge now, so I will go to a hotel. I'm sorry we had to argue like this on today of all days, but it seems it's how we're destined to be. I will call you in a week or two."

Utterly exhausted and wrung out with emotion, Kallie didn't try to stop her and when she heard her mother's car roar away up the lane she poured herself a glass of wine and curled up on the settee, frowning to see she had laddered her black tights. Her eyelids felt heavy and she hoped she would sleep later, for she knew she needed to rest. She took a sip then raised her glass in a toast.

"I hope you didn't hear all that! Here's to you, Gran and Grandad, the most wonderful grandparents a girl could ever have wished for. I love you and I'm happy that you're together. I'll be okay, I promise."

Chapter 5

ALISTAIR
Australia, 2014

"Good morning, Alistair! How are we doing today? Need anything?"

"I don't know how you are, darling girl, or if you need anything, but I'm dying and no thank you!" Alistair raised his head from the pillow and said, with a twinkle in his eye and only half-joking. "Unless you can give me something to hasten things along a little? You're all wonderful but it's very boring being stuck in here and I have it on good authority that it's just great on the Other Side!"

The young nurse tilted her head and wagged her finger in a 'now don't be naughty' gesture before tucking the sheets tighter around him, much to his irritation. He didn't want to be fussed over by anyone, never had. He just wanted to be left in private until his damaged lungs stopped taking in oxygen and his struggling heart stopped beating and then what? He'd never thought about it until now, not really.

He'd experienced many dangerous situations because of his love of adventure, would even go so far as to say he'd come face to face with death a couple of times, up front and personal, but he had never considered what might come afterwards. He'd never talked about such matters to anyone. His friends were all like him, gung-ho and willing to face their fears head on and hang the consequences. All he'd wanted, he now realised, was a swift death, preferably while on one of his wild escapades. He certainly wasn't enjoying this prolonged passing, and appreciated for the first time just how much his younger brother Finlay had had to endure almost twenty-five years ago.

That brought him to reflecting on his nephew, his 'good authority' on the Afterlife. Alex had an unshakeable belief in life after death and made no bones about letting people know about it.

Alistair hadn't seen his nephew in years and years, since Alex was nine years old and Alistair had gone home to Scotland for Finlay's funeral. He had fond memories of the happy, skinny little kid whose dad had died, yet who claimed to be able to see and talk to him any time he wanted. It had been disconcerting to watch how the little chap had conducted himself so confidently as his father had been buried, his little face serious as he looked up at his mother, reassuring her that his daddy was just fine in heaven.

And now he was a well-known psychic medium with his own TV show, no less. Alex's mum, who to Alistair's delighted surprise and appreciation sent a card with a news-packed letter and photographs every Christmas since Alistair had settled in Australia and finally had a fixed address, had emailed him about it and sent him a link to an episode of the programme. When Alistair got around to watching it, he'd sat shaking his head in bafflement at what his handsome nephew could apparently do. But was it real? He didn't know, though of course to say it couldn't be real was to say that Alex was some kind of fraudster.

Alex had written a book too, but Alistair hadn't read it as

he preferred direct action to sitting glued to the printed word, so never read anything unless he had to, not even maps when he was exploring regions that were new to him.

The nurse went out of the room and did not close the door behind her, even though he must have asked a dozen times for it to be kept closed. He especially didn't want it open at visiting time; he didn't want to hear the comings and goings of other patients' visitors as there would be none for him.

No-one even knew he was in here. But that's the decision he'd made, because he didn't want his mates coming here and seeing him like this; weak and sick and vulnerable. And he certainly didn't want to burden Alex and Alex's mum, Aileen, the only family he had, with the faff and expense of travelling ten thousand miles just to watch him die and then bury him.

"Quite right. It's an awfully long way, and they wouldn't make it in time anyway."

What the hell?

Alistair's eyes darted wildly round the room, but there was no-one there. He listened hard, thinking he must be able to hear conversation from people going past his room, or a television or radio blaring from a neighbouring room.

"If you look to your left and just relax your eyes you'll be able to see me."

Alistair went totally still. The soft Scottish accent he now realised he was hearing in his mind rather than with his ears was unmistakable, but did he really recognise that voice after so many years? He counted under his breath to ten and then turned his head with a slow, reluctant motion.

At first, he saw nothing but the print on the wall, Monet's 'Wild Poppies' the label on the frame said, but as he narrowed his eyes and stared, an outline of a person began to form. At first it was so faint he could still make out the Monet as if viewing it through a haze of smoke, but the figure shimmered and gradually grew more solid and Alistair's jaw dropped as he found himself staring at his younger brother.

The brother who had died over two decades ago.

Alistair reached the peak of loud and colourful swearing just as the nurse bustled back in with a syringe and a medicine cup containing his daily dose of pills on a flat metal tray. Shocked, she looked at him with raised eyebrows, asking if he was in pain.

Dragging his eyes from what he was certain must be a drug-induced hallucination, even though it had been hours since his last dose of medication, he apologised for his bad language.

"Tell her you've got cramp in your leg."

Unable to think coherently Alistair obediently repeated the words, while pointing to his left leg.

"Want me to massage it for you?"

Before he could object, the sheets were stripped back and the nurse was asking whether it was thigh or calf that needed attention.

The hallucination chuckled. *"Say it's both. You might as well delay having the medications, they won't do you any good."*

Alistair scrutinised the nurse's kind, deeply tanned face to see if she'd heard his brother speaking, but she was patiently waiting for him to tell her where the cramp was. Not sure what to say he pretended to wince while sweeping his hand to indicate that his whole leg hurt. She murmured words of sympathy and reassurance as she rolled up his pyjama trousers and got to work on his calf muscle with strong, expert fingers.

At first, he rather enjoyed it, but then he realised he was

starting to feel peculiar. Extremely peculiar. His body was slowly but most definitely going numb, the sensation creeping like an icy fog from the feet upwards. He could no longer feel the nurse's hands on his leg. He looked down. Yes, she was still massaging away with both hands working in a smooth, circular motion around his knee. He moved his eyes to his own hands, fingers interlaced, palms flat on top of his distended stomach, but he could not feel the fabric of his pyjama jacket or the warmth of his skin beneath.

Pinprick black and silver dots flashed in the periphery of his vision and a low hissing sound began in his ears, like air leaking from a tyre. His pulse sped up until the hissing sound was drowned out by the wild thrumming of his heart, increasing his fear as its erratic rhythm registered in his brain. Whatever was going on in his body, he knew it wasn't good.

So, was this it? Was this his last hour, his final few moments as Alistair Donald Kelburn, adventurer and explorer?

Unbidden, his mind flooded with memories of the life he had lived, his birth to present time fully remembered in every detail. Not the life-flashing-before-the-eyes like a film on fast forward that you've heard about, but life in its entirety known all in one precise moment.

Certain elements stood out and he studied them in wonder: his initial jealousy when Finlay was born and needed the almost constant attention of their mother, soon countered by their fierce and mutual brotherly love as they grew up together; the bewilderment of his first day at school; his troubled teen years; the quest for ways that would satisfy his constant need for the adrenalin rush that only danger could bring.

His travels around the world and choosing to settle in Australia having found the place where the surfing, diving, sailing, climbing and all the other pursuits he had wholeheartedly and often dangerously embraced were second to none; all the jobs he'd taken to earn enough money to pay his bills, from tending bar to shearing sheep; his all-consuming grief when he heard that Fin had died and the guilt and frustration he'd felt during the interminable journey from South America to get back home; the disbelief on hearing the diagnosis of the disease that was killing him now, most likely caused by his many years of heavy smoking and drinking.

Hundreds, thousands of memories flooded his brain, and he was grateful that the good kind far outnumbered the bad. He'd had a wonderful life, just wonderful, and he felt that he had led it well, daring to venture out into the big wide world and experience as much as he could while doing harm to nothing and no-one.

He'd thought he was ready, now he had the indignities and pain of failing liver and lungs to contend with, to leave it all. But now he'd had this weird and wonderful replay of his vigorous life at what he suspected was the point of no return, he found himself rather attached to it and wished he could recover his good health and get back to doing all the things he loved.

He was only in his sixties and there was so much more he'd hoped to do before shuffling off into the sunset. His ramshackle but much-loved beach house was in the middle of renovations. A sailing trip was planned with his buddies (actually more drinking than sailing, but that was what it was all about, right?). There were still planes to jump out of, wild seas to dive beneath, sheer rock faces to climb and conquer.

He'd been thinking of getting in touch with Mandu to arrange a month-long camp-out with his wise and funny friend who knew all there was to know about survival in the Outback. He'd always thought he'd go home to Scotland again one day, revisit old haunts under happier circumstances than his last visit for Fin's funeral, but he knew now that, provided his last wishes were carried out, only his ashes would return there.

Was that him making that terrible rasping noise? Were those tears of self-pity rolling from his eyes?

The pillow was suddenly whipped from beneath his head while the nurse simultaneously hit a red button on the call panel above his bed, jolting him back to the present crisis.

"Mr Kelburn! Mr Kelburn! Can you hear me?"

"They'll try everything to get you back because that's what they're trained to do, but we all must die eventually and your time, brother, has come. Just relax and let go. There's nothing to be afraid of."

He could clearly hear the words of both voices, his brother and the nurse, even though one was an amused whisper and the other a frantic shout. All hell broke loose then as a doctor, white jacket flying, came crashing in, followed closely by two more nurses, one pulling and one pushing the emergency cart.

It was like an invasion, not only of his small, clinical room but also of his body. They talked with urgent voices in a code meaningless to him as they ripped open his pyjama jacket, careless of the buttons that tore away and rolled under the bed. The doctor started compressing Alistair's chest, a nurse stuck pads on him and yet another put an oxygen mask over his face. The nurse that had called the crash team stood by the defibrillator waiting for it to charge. He could see and hear all this, and he braced himself for the surge of electricity that would soon be racing through his skin and muscle and rib cage to his labouring heart.

His body jumped, arching and lifting from the bed.

"Again!" Someone barked. "Again!"

Suspended in that place between somewhere and elsewhere another memory came blasting into his mind as each surge of electricity jolted his body. A memory so long buried because he had had to force it deep or go mad with grief. He really had not thought about it, about her, for decades.

He tested the name in his mind for a moment, almost tasting it as a sweetness counteracting the metallic taste on his tongue. He delved deep to bring her heart-shaped face to his mind's eye, her huge, deep brown eyes that glowed with intelligence and humour and the charming dimples in both cheeks that appeared as she talked, smiled and laughed. She'd had a face that warned of mischief, and he'd fallen for her the first time he'd met her.

Jeanie.

Jeanie, who had left this earth far too young and too soon in a tragic climbing accident, but Alistair knew she'd far rather go that way than the way he was going. Better to die quickly doing something you love, they and their like-minded friends had said often.

She had been the love of his life, more of a daredevil and thrill seeker than even he had been until this illness forced him to a stop. No woman since, and there had been many, had ever matched up to her, so he had given up looking for someone he could wholeheartedly commit to and spent his life a bachelor.

Surprised that remembering her didn't bring the unbearable pain as he'd long suspected it would, it occurred to him that he felt nothing at all. But he could see and hear everything. How could that be? How could he be watching all this happen as if he were a spectator in the room?

And then he realised that a spectator was, in fact, exactly what he had become, because he was no longer in his body. He was standing next to his little brother, who was grinning at him with pure joy written all over his face.

***

Alex dialled his mother's number, prepared to wait as she'd most likely be doing some knitting or cross stitch or one of her other many creative hobbies, but she answered before it had barely begun to ring. Her soft Scottish voice brought a smile to Alex's face.

"Hi Mum. That was quick!"

She chuckled. "Well, as it happens, I was about to call you."

"Oh?"

"But why are you ringing me, you don't usually call at this time of the day?"

He sighed, not sure how she'd take the news that Uncle Alistair had died. They hadn't seen him in years, in fact since Alex's father's funeral, but she was a sensitive soul, easily moved to tears. When he told her, though, she didn't get upset, but asked him how and when Alistair had died and how Alex had learned of it. There was something in her voice that made him glad that he'd prepared an outright lie about how he'd known.

"Liver and lung cancer, undoubtedly caused by his crazy lifestyle. He had my name and phone number as his main contact, so the hospital rang me. There's nothing for us to do though, as regards his funeral, because he left explicit instructions for us not to fly over there. He's going to be cremated and he wants his ashes to be buried in Scotland, preferably with Dad, if you have no objection."

There was a long silence, and Alex pictured his diminutive mother reaching out to straighten the picture of the long haired Highland cow on the wall, or fiddle with the pen that was always on the notepad in case she had to write anything down.

"Alex," she said eventually. "I appreciate why you aren't telling me the truth, but the fact is I'd not long finished speaking to someone from the hospital, as Alistair had given my name to contact as we have stayed in touch all these years. I was given the name and number of his solicitor so I could learn what his wishes were, but I haven't yet made the call. So, as you know so much, am I to assume that you have been communicating with your father? Are they together?"

Hearing the warmth in her voice Alex was relieved that she was keeping a sense of humour about that aspect of his life that she said she'd never truly understand. She especially couldn't understand how Finlay was Alex's constant guide and helper, but he replied that they were, indeed, together.

"Dad went to him a little while before he passed over and was with him when it finally happened. Alistair didn't suffer, it was quick, and he was just amazed at how easy it all was and that Dad was actually there. They're going to have a high old time catching up, and I'm delighted, even though it means I might have to work without Dad for a while."

After talking some more about Fin and Alistair, and what might need to be done to bring Alistair's ashes home, they caught up on other news. Aileen informed him that Frank had taken up lawn bowls, which made Alex chuckle at the image he had of his notoriously competitive stepfather playing what Alex imagined to be a rather genteel game.

Alex told his mother that Beth was enjoying her job and also loving her training to become a bereavement counsellor, that his engineering business was doing well and he was still waiting to hear if a new series of his television show would be commissioned.

"Are we likely to see you and Beth this side of Christmas?" his mother asked, laughter tinkling in her voice.

He ended the call with a promise that he and Beth would get up to Scotland to see her and Frank at the earliest opportunity.

Part Three

LIFE, DEATH AND IN BETWEEN
2015

Chapter 6

"Well done, Paul! A beautiful ceremony and a wonderful reception, and everyone enjoyed your speech. I was beginning to think you'd never marry, you know."

He laughed, his whole face lighting up in a way Sylvia loved to see.

"Nor me, Gran. Any woman has a lot to live up to thanks to my having such gorgeous and amazing ladies in the family, but I've found myself a beauty, haven't I?"

He certainly had. Adele was a delightful young woman, and Sylvia suspected, the first to really steal her grandson's heart. Even the lovely girl he'd been engaged to a few years back had not been able to bring such tangible joy to Paul's life. Adele had calmed him a little and managed to pull him gently away from being a total workaholic who lived, breathed and ate celebrity business deals, and he was all the happier for it.

Sylvia smiled at the way Paul's face softened as he switched his gaze from her to his new bride, who was across the room talking to her parents. Adele had chosen a simple, fitted, very elegant cream gown for her wedding dress, and wore no jewellery other than a scattering of tiny diamond pins in her short dark hair to complement those in her bouquet of cream and pale apricot roses and her beautiful diamond engagement ring. Would they have children and make her and Simon great-grandparents again, Sylvia asked herself? If they did, how would Beth and Alex cope with that? Especially Beth?

No, no Sylvia, she admonished herself. *Don't go down that road.*

She hugged Paul and told him how devastatingly handsome he looked before moving away in search of the other members of her family. She spotted Beth and Alex talking to Adele's sister, Lily, but where was Simon?

She scanned the room, looking for the long, rangy form of her husband, knowing when she found him that he would be running his finger inside his collar or pulling irritably at his cravat.

Paul had insisted on the men being kitted out in top hat and tails with wing collared shirts and fancy waistcoats, and Simon's loud and sometimes furious objections had been firmly overridden by everyone. When she'd finally seen him in the full get-up she'd thought he looked wonderful. Well, except for the hat. When he'd plonked that on his head the tops of his ears had folded downward beneath the brim and she'd had to stifle a giggle or risk setting him off on another rant.

She located Simon with a knot of people she didn't recognise standing in front of a beautiful arched window. He and all the other men had ditched the top hats at the first opportunity, but sure enough he was tugging at his clothes. If he wasn't adjusting the collar or fiddling with the cravat, just as she'd imagined, he was tugging the embroidered waistcoat down at the front.

As she neared him she could see how he gazed straight over the head of the much shorter man he was in conversation with, a blank expression on his face. Was he merely bored by his companion, or was it something else, something she needed to worry about?

Feeling her heart skip a beat, Sylvia moved swiftly to rescue the situation.

"Hello, darling. I'm in need of a drink, would you mind going to find me one please? A glass of Champagne would be lovely."

He barely seemed to acknowledge her but moved off to do as she asked. Sylvia fastened her brightest smile onto her face and introduced herself to the man as, "Sylvia-grandmother-of-the-groom."

She didn't know him but took in at a glance the artfully spiked hair, the air of supreme confidence, and gosh, was that make-up on his face, mascara on his lashes? His lips were suspiciously glossy too. From the make-up and the rather dazzling sheen of his hair, face and clothes, Sylvia could be sure that he was a showbiz type, so very likely he was a client of Paul's.

There were a lot of them here, quite a few recognisable TV and film personalities, and for that reason just one reporter and one photographer, professionals Paul knew and trusted, had been invited to cover the event. To protect the famous, and even the not-so-famous, other guests had been asked not to take photographs on this occasion, with the promise of free copies of the professional ones in due course. Sylvia suspected that any photos featuring the showbiz stars were destined for a society magazine for some great fee.

She made small talk, not at all surprised to find that the man was indeed rather boring, definitely self-centred, until it dawned on her that Simon was not coming back with her drink.

"My husband's been waylaid, I think. I'd better go and find

him, I really do want that drink. Lovely to talk to you. Enjoy the rest of the reception."

The man courteously bowed his head to her, probably as relieved as she was to bring an end to their stilted conversation, and strolled away from her as she tried to guess where Simon might have got to.

For weeks and weeks she had worried about this day, how Simon would behave. Was she right to suspect that something was wrong with him, or was it just a blip and she was making mountains out of molehills? Sure, he had moments of forgetfulness, but didn't everyone have that from time to time? Especially as one got older. It hadn't worried her unduly at first, just caused a little irritation now and again, but he was constantly forgetting appointments, names and phone numbers. His moods were erratic, and the displays of temper certainly unusual. And then he'd worry and obsess over silly little things, like did he have his wallet in his pocket, or was she sure she had locked all the doors before coming to bed? There were moments, just a second or two, when he seemed completely blank, as if he didn't know where he was or, even more alarming, who she was.

But he was eighty-four, six years older than her. Was it just old age? He had always been energetic, with a terrific brain, absorbing like a sponge and remembering with accuracy the knowledge contained in all the non-fiction books he read. He had several hobbies that required planning and manual dexterity. She'd tried to convince herself that the changes in him were caused by having too much on his mind, too many things going on—after all, they were almost as busy even this far into his retirement as they had been when he'd been working.

And, she had to admit, though the sudden death of their

little great-granddaughter had stunned them all, Simon had found it extremely hard accepting that Beth, in deep mourning for the loss of her beautiful baby, had separated from Alex and moved back in with her parents. Sylvia and Simon had such a row about it, she still smarted to think about it.

It had started with Simon shouting, "What is our daughter thinking in letting her daughter walk out on her marriage? What about poor Alex? He's grieving over Amber too, isn't he? A wife's place is beside her husband no matter what the circumstance, so Beth should be at home with Alex."

Sylvia had countered by saying she felt they ought to support Beth, a grieving mother, until she could think straight again.

"Who knows what goes on inside a marriage, Simon, except the two who are in it? I understand what you're saying, but I don't want you saying anything to her other than you love her and want what's best for her."

From there it had escalated, with Sylvia only slowly comprehending that Simon's anger at Beth was his way of venting his own grief at the loss of dear little Amber, but when she'd said this he'd stormed off to his workshop. She was relieved at his going, though, as it meant he would take out his frustration on some inanimate object rather than her.

But she'd wondered herself why Beth had walked out on Alex. Of course, they had no knowledge of other factors within their marriage which might have contributed to the break up, and she would not pry. She just thanked the heavens that they were back together and seemed very happy, both for their sake and because their reconciliation had restored Simon's good temper.

Though the whole family deeply mourned baby Amber, who hadn't even lived to see her first birthday, they got on with their lives, for what choice did they have? Sylvia had been relieved to get settled back into their routine, and then Paul's announcement last year that he was getting married had been a delightful surprise that had lifted everyone's spirits.

Well, everyone except Simon, once he'd been told it was to be a wedding with all the bells and whistles, not only the morning suits for the men, but also big hats and fancy dresses for the ladies, a five-star venue for the ceremony and reception, a seven-course wedding banquet, and so on and so on.

Sylvia had been thrilled at the idea of such a grand event, knowing that with Adele's innate good taste, Paul's PR skills and business contacts, and the likelihood of Adele's wealthy father footing some if not all of the expense, it would be a beautiful and memorable wedding.

She, Anna and Beth had spent a few happy days hunting down their outfits and she'd looked forward to showing what she'd chosen to Simon. Unfortunately, he had marred things slightly for her by going into an almighty strop because of the amount she had spent and the reminder that he was required to hire his morning suit from a very expensive gentlemen's outfitter. Yes, Sylvia acknowledged, she knew he preferred to always be dressed in casual, comfy clothes, but surely one day in a tail coat wouldn't kill him! Paul had offered to foot the bill, so surely her splashing out on a special dress with matching coat, shoes, handbag and hat wasn't that bad!

He'd accepted grudgingly that her new clothes were gorgeous but had gone on and on about the morning suit for days, until Sylvia had finally lost her temper and told him in no uncertain terms that he would wear the coat, the striped trousers, the fancy waistcoat, the shiny shoes, hat, starched shirt and even red silk underpants if their grandson required it, and she would not hear another word about it. And she hadn't. He'd simply closed his mouth with an audible snap, compressed his lips into a bloodless straight line, and not uttered a single word of protest about it since.

All through the fittings at the very fancy hire place and even getting dressed this morning he'd not complained, but she'd almost prefer it if he had muttered his quiet obscenities, because for quite a while it had been as if he'd shut himself away from her and become unreachable. And all over a suit!

Sylvia was brought back to the present by Beth's arrival at her side. She smiled with loving warmth at her granddaughter, who looked gorgeous in a cherry red dress, topped with a beautiful cream hat adorned with cream silk flowers that wound round the crown and spilled onto the brim. There were fine lines around her eyes now, but at least her smile reached her eyes these days. She was still far too thin in Sylvia's opinion, though Beth promised everyone she ate healthy food and plenty of it.

"Having fun, darling? I'm looking for your Grandad."

"Pops is outside talking to Mum and Dad, and Alex has just gone over to join them. The men all look so handsome in their get-up, don't they? When I saw Alex it took my breath away!" She laughed as she said, "Until he put the hat on. I bet Pops hates it? Dad and Alex certainly do, and I know the minute we get home Alex will pull on his tattiest jeans and raggiest rugby shirt."

"Yes, and Simon will change into his usual comfy trousers and checked shirt. Do you know, I've hardly ever seen him in anything else since he retired? He always wore suits and ties when he was working, so handsome! But now it's casual every single day, no matter what we're doing. Open his wardrobe and that's all you see, dark trousers and checked shirts. And all his belts and shoes are brown."

"Well, I suppose it makes getting dressed easier! Shall we go and join them?"

Sylvia took Beth's proffered arm and they strolled out onto the grand terrace that ran the full width of the magnificent hotel. Stone steps, curved and sweeping, perfect for the official wedding photographs, led down onto manicured gardens of stunning flower beds and emerald green lawns mown and rolled into stripes. There were about a dozen pretty, beribboned awnings dotted about, sheltering white-clothed tables from the sun, laid out with canapés, exotic sweets, party favours, cocktails and drinks of all kinds.

Anna, Felix, Simon and Alex were in front of the bar housed in a grand marquee, Simon holding a half-full pint glass of beer and a full flute of Champagne, so Sylvia was happy to think he had at least had the intention of returning to her with the drink she'd asked for.

She curled her arm round his waist, mindful of the wide, feathered brim of her hat bumping against his arm.

"There you are! Is that for me?" She took the glass and sipped. "Mmm, heaven. Isn't it just the perfect day?"

Simon had clutched the glass for a little too long so the bubbly drink was no longer ice-cold as she preferred it, but no matter. She wouldn't ask him to change it for a fresh one.

She beamed round at her beloved close-knit family, but she hadn't missed the look of puzzlement on Alex's face before he'd seen her approach and gathered himself to smile at her. What had Simon being saying to him? Or what had Alex seen in Simon? Her grandson-in-law spooked Sylvia a bit, because of what he did. She didn't quite understand it, she wasn't even sure she believed in it—she'd watched his TV show with a mixture of disbelief and awe and she'd read his autobiography—but, whether it was due to his having psychic powers or not, she knew with certainty that he was unusually sharp and perceptive about people.

Now, however, with Anna and Beth in earshot, was not the time to ask him, and she hoped Alex wouldn't say anything to Beth later if he had any concerns about Simon. Beth would be sure to tell Anna, as she shared everything with her mum, and at all costs Sylvia wanted to protect her daughter and granddaughter, especially her granddaughter, for as long as she could if it turned out that Simon had the illness she was more and more suspecting he had.

Beth was a strong woman in many ways, incredibly so, but Sylvia knew there was also a fragility in her that had always been there and could easily rise to the surface again under pressure.

During the months Beth had lived with her parents, Anna and Felix, after Amber had died and she'd separated from Alex, Sylvia had seen and despaired of her vulnerable state and the depression she descended into. Yes, Beth was grieving for her baby, and everyone knew that would take forever and a day, but she had somehow got it into her head that she was not worthy of Alex, which added to her sense of profound grief and loss.

When Alex had at last confronted her and finally sorted it all out, Sylvia had been so relieved. But still, you never got over a bereavement of that nature. No parent should have to bury a child, nor should any generation have to bury one of a younger generation.

Beth and Alex truly loved each other, she could see that, but there were times she found herself wondering if they'd managed to repair their relationship so it was unbreakable in the face of any further trouble or tragedy, fervently hoping that it was as secure as it seemed to be. These worries about her family were always bubbling under the surface in her mind, and that, she knew, was the burden carried the moment one became a parent.

Come on Sylvia, she warned herself. *Stop it now or you'll be crying.*

A loud hand bell started clanging. People stopped their conversations mid-sentence and turned as one towards the source of the sound, wondering what it might mean. A man, a town crier no less, in full livery of long red coat with gold braiding, white shirt with elaborately frilled cuffs, buckled shoes polished to a mirror shine, and black tricorn hat with a large white ostrich feather on it, strode among them, ringing his bell and exhorting everyone to go inside as the newlyweds were preparing to leave.

Careful of their slender high heels sinking into the grass, Sylvia, Anna and Beth linked arms and walked ahead of their husbands to join the others gathering beneath the chandeliers of the room where the reception had been.

All the tables and chairs and been cleared away and Paul and Adele were standing hand in hand on a low platform at the far end, dressed now to go straight to Heathrow airport for their flight to a one-month safari honeymoon in Kenya.

Sylvia found herself next to Adele's mother, an elegant but rather glacial woman, and said how lovely, happy and radiant Adele looked.

Once the newlyweds had left in a dark grey limousine trailing tin cans tied to the back bumper with white ribbons, Sylvia said to Simon it was time they went home. The party would continue until late with a disco and live band taking turns to entertain, with some of the guests—those that could afford the five-star prices—staying overnight in the hotel, breakfasting in style the next morning before returning to real life.

She and Simon had the choice to stay the night but as the grand country hotel was less than an hour from their own home, they'd decided they'd prefer to wake up in their own bed the next morning.

It took a long time to extract themselves as there were so many people they needed to say goodbye to, so it was a relief to finally climb into the back of the chauffeur-driven silver Mercedes that Paul had arranged as their transport for the day.

Sylvia kicked off her shoes, flexed her toes, and leaned her head back with a tired but contented sigh. Taking Simon's hand, she said, "I bet you can't wait to get that suit off, darling, and return it and that ridiculous hat to the hire shop."

He slowly swung his head towards her and she felt alarm grip her insides at the glazed look in his eyes. "What are you talking about? What hat?"

Sylvia realised then that he'd left the hat at the hotel and she'd have to call as soon as they got home to make sure someone retrieved it. But more concerning than that, far more worrying, was the blank expression on Simon's face.

Chapter 7

A long, flatbed truck blocked the entry to his engineering works when Alex drove up, so he parked round the side of the building and walked back to watch it being unloaded. It was a delivery of steel and other metals for a number of jobs they had on the go, and Alex enjoyed the shouts and banter of the men as they unloaded and organised where the heavy, unwieldy material was to go.

When the fun was over and the lorry had backed out and away with a trailing cloud of black smoke from its exhaust, he strolled through to the office to be greeted by Trish. She had not long joined the firm as a part-time administrator, hired by Alex's manager to run the office and deal with all the paperwork.

"We're getting busier, boss," Bill had said to Alex. "And we're behind with the invoicing. Dave says his wife has relevant experience and is looking for a part-time job, so I think we should call her in. Now you're so busy with other matters we really do need someone dedicated to the paperwork, keeping track and making sure the invoices are paid on time. It'll be worth it, Alex, trust me."

Alex had inwardly smiled at Bill's 'other matters' knowing he was quite bemused about what it was that kept Alex away from his own factory so much these days. He decided to make himself a mug of tea before tracking Bill down and having a general walkabout with him so he could be updated on the latest orders.

The little kitchen was still a shock to the eyes and nose, not because of the state it was in but because of the state it *wasn't* in. He always expected to see unwashed mugs and used teaspoons everywhere including some piled up untidily in the sink, spilled coffee powder, grains of sugar and puddles of milk on the worktops and on the floor. On top of that, the whiff of an old, much-used dishcloth left wet and balled up for too long. He'd suggested they go to plastic cups and spoons but the outcry had soon put paid to that one, so the large, thick mugs and metal spoons had stayed, along with the mess.

But there was no mess on the days Trish was in. On finding out that she was regularly washing up and cleaning the kitchen, even taking it upon herself to bring in clean tea towels and take the used ones home to launder, Alex had gathered Bill and the five other men who worked in the factory and told them that he did not want her doing this.

"Wash up your own things," he'd said. "And use the paper towels provided to dry your mugs. Trish is here to do the invoicing and make sure you get your wages paid on time, she is not here to clean up after you."

No-one had taken any notice, and Alex knew that they still left it for her to do, and of course she did it without complaint. He sighed as he chucked a tea bag in a mug, a mug that didn't even have brown stains in the bottom of it any longer, and filled it with hot water from the dispenser. He was stirring in a splash of milk when Trish appeared in the doorway.

She hesitated, as if not sure whether to come all the way in. From the beginning Alex had sensed she held herself back, as if she was a little nervous of him, and he could think of a few reasons that might be. For one thing, he was the boss. But, the real reason for her slight agitation in his presence was the same as Bill's and all the other members of staff: it was the fact that he was a psychic medium. That made a lot of people nervous.

He smiled at her. "You still clean up in here, don't you?"

She gave a rueful, slightly apologetic grin. "I really don't mind. The guys are busy, and of course their hands are always dirty because of the jobs they do. I know they appreciate it," she laughed. "And I really can't stand an untidy kitchen! Please don't worry about it. At least they keep the toilet clean now they know I have to use it!"

Alex laughed, knowing she was right, and who tidied up the kitchen was a battle he shouldn't even try to win.

"Well, thank you. I certainly appreciate it, it's nice being able to make a drink without worrying if I'm going to get salmonella or something equally nasty. I hear you're doing a great job for us, I hope you're enjoying it?"

She nodded, saying that she had a lot of fun because all the men were so friendly and funny. They looked after her really well, she said.

"Bill told me that you volunteer at Rainstones House?" Alex said. "I've been there a couple of times. The staff there are very open minded and invite me along at the request of patients who want the kind of reassurance they feel I can give. What do you do there?"

"I help out in the hospice Day Patient Unit once a week. It's basically meeting and greeting guests, making refreshments, helping out with whatever entertainment has been laid on. Such a wonderful place, I really enjoy it."

Alex sensed her hesitation and knew there was more. She dropped her gaze and said, "My half-sister died in the hospice and my father's in the dementia wing."

He had a vague sense of someone with her, and it was confirmed when he heard in his mind *'pat-a-cake,'* spoken in the vaguest of whispers. He tried to focus on whoever it was, thinking it could be her sister offering a game she and Trish had played when they were little to help identify her, but the link was too weak.

Dismissing it, he said, "Oh, I'm so sorry. That must be very hard for you."

"Losing my sister was hard. My father was diagnosed with Alzheimer's in his eighties and he's a hundred and one next month." She laughed at the look on Alex's face. "I'm a product of his third marriage and he was nearly sixty when I came along. Shall I tell Bill you're here?"

"I already know!" Bill's booming voice rang out just before his rotund frame filled the door widthways, trapping Trish in the kitchen. "Hey there, boss, how are you? How was the wedding of the year? We all want to see pics of you in the monkey suit!"

Seeing Trish's puzzled expression, Bill explained that Alex's brother-in-law had recently got married and that there had been quite a few famous faces amongst the guests. He winked at Alex. "Including our Alex, eh boss?"

Trish smiled uncertainly, and muttered that she had to get back to work. She sidled past Bill, who had stepped back to give her room, and Alex watched her go to her tidy and dust-free desk, grabbing the phone almost before it started to ring.

Bill said, "She's an absolute bloody Godsend, Alex, you've no idea. The invoices are up to date, she chases late orders and payments like a terrier, taking no shit from anybody. And she keeps this bloody room clean and disinfected, as you can see!"

"And she keeps the swearing down, I hope."

Bill laughed, his jowls and big beer belly wobbling. "Yes, there is less of the bad language when she's around, I must admit. Now then, let me bring you up to date. And the first thing I have to tell you is, Clive is leaving us."

"What? Why?"

"He and his missus have decided to retire and move closer to family. He's our longest serving member of staff so we'll need to give him a merry old send off. But don't worry, Trish is on the case and she's going to put an ad in the paper and help us find a replacement. It'll be a month or two before Clive moves, and I'm certain we can keep on top of the orders even without him in the short term."

Pleased that his factory was in the capable hands of Bill, Alex followed him round while he gave a running commentary on the jobs being worked on, reflecting for the thousandth time as he listened to Bill how much he missed being here on a day to day basis. It was his business after all, he'd started it and was still the sole owner, and he loved it. But the TV show had brought recognition beyond his wildest dreams and taken him to a point where he was constantly in demand and just couldn't be here full-time any more. That's why he'd promoted Bill to factory manager, knowing he'd do a great job of keeping the place running efficiently and ensuring that the reputation of Kelburn Engineering and the goods they produced remained high.

He inhaled the familiar smells of hot metals and oils while

casting his eyes around the bays where projects ranging from utilitarian sheet metal work to ornate spiral staircases and everything in between were being made by his highly-skilled team. The high-ceilinged factory rang with the ringing, buzzing, hissing sounds of hammers on steel, heavy duty band saws, grinders and drills and welding equipment, making Alex long to grab some gear and get his hands dirty doing something. Anything. But with Bill managing the factory, a great team making the goods, and Trish so efficiently running the administration side of things, he really wasn't needed here.

Tour over and satisfied that all was well, in fact very well indeed, Alex decided to go home to Beth. She would be back from work by the time he reached the house, and he thought he could get some paperwork cleared and then the two of them could to go out for dinner.

The drive home took him through the village and past the road where he'd lived during his and Beth's painful separation, and he was delighted to see his old neighbour Maisie Fanshawe walking along the village High Street, a bag of shopping carried in each hand. He smiled to see the dyed gingery hair on her head and the pristine white trainers on her feet, their fat red laces tied in a double bow. He pulled over and offered her a lift back.

"Oh, Alex! How lovely to see you. Yes please, these bags are a bit heavy. Jack's out with friends, so he won't be home; he'll be so sorry to miss you."

She got into the car, heaving her shopping bags into the foot well in front of her.

"How is Jack, Maisie?"

"Oh, no better, no worse. But how are you, how's Beth? Oh, we do miss you living so close. And what about your TV show, Alex? Is there going to be another one? I tell everyone I meet that I know you personally and how wonderful you are!"

Laughing, Alex thanked her. She was a lovely lady with a disabled husband who had befriended him when he'd been alone and hurting, and his next-door neighbours, Lily and Scott Miller, who were expecting their first baby at the time, had also become his friends.

He recalled with a shudder the incredible shock felt by everyone when Scott had died. Both he and Alex had been hit by an out of control van while they were out for a run. Losing Scott just before their baby was born had been terrible. There were a lot of memories packed into this part of town.

As was her way, Maisie was still chatting away as Alex pulled up outside her house, so he switched off the engine and turned so he could look at her. She tended to switch from subject to subject very quickly, requiring her listeners to concentrate or lose the thread very quickly.

Now she was saying, "I hear Adele got married to Beth's brother, how amazing is that? I well remember how she'd looked at him when she first saw him! Lily's away at her parents' villa with her daughter Hope, did you know? Oh, of course you'd know, Lily went to the wedding didn't she!" Maisie laughed at herself.

Alex said that Lily had very much enjoyed herself at the wedding and he and Beth had promised to visit her as soon as she was home again.

Maisie, her face suddenly falling, said, "That girl does miss her husband so. What a tragic accident that was, and you so close to death too. Are you fully recovered from the accident, Alex?" Without waiting for an answer, she pointed back to the place that Alex had lived.

It had been a very run-down semi that a friend had let him have for a low rent because he was going to do it up as soon as he'd finished another couple of building projects. It was all done now and looked smart with its new windows, paintwork and neat front garden.

"Did you ever see inside it when it was done up by your builder friend?"

"Yes, he invited me and Beth to see it before he put it on the market." Seeing Maisie's expression he assured her that they had knocked on her door to see if she wanted to have a look too but she and Jack had been out, and continued, "The transformation is stunning. We were tempted, but really the place holds too few fond memories for either of us so we decided not to make an offer on it. And I'm glad we didn't; we love the house we're living in now. Anyway, Maisie, let me carry those bags in for you and then I must be on my way."

Maisie's hand flew to her mouth. "Oh, and here's me rabbiting on and not even offering you a cup of tea. I can manage the bags, Alex, but will you promise to bring Beth to see us soon? Jack would love to see you both."

Alex made the promise and drove the rest of the way home, searching out Beth as soon as he arrived. She was in the kitchen, standing in front of the open fridge door.

"Hot flush?" he quipped.

"Oh, ha-ha, but I'll have you know I've got many years to go before you can legitimately make a remark like that! How come you're back from the factory so early?"

"Well now, the sad fact is I'm not needed at my own business these days, so I thought I'd come home where my qualities are still appreciated by my beautiful wife. I would have been home sooner but I gave Maisie a lift home, she'd been shopping in the village."

Laughing, she said, "I bet she talked your ears off. Are she and Jack well? We must go and see them soon. Now, what shall we have for supper?"

Alex said he wanted to take her out.

"Ooh, lovely! Have you booked somewhere?"

He shook his head. "I'll do it now. Anywhere you particularly fancy?"

Beth said she didn't mind where they went, then had second thoughts and named a place a colleague at work had recently mentioned to her as a good place to eat. It was a little Italian bistro, tucked away up a side street in the town, with checked tablecloths, candles stuck into wax-covered Chianti bottles, cheerful service and good, wholesome food.

"Sounds perfect. I'll find the number and book us a table. It's a lovely evening, so as soon as I'm done with some paperwork let's go into town, have a walk along the canal and a drink in the Old Bear before dinner."

He ambled into the little downstairs room they both used as an office, where a quick online search took him to the website of the restaurant. He dialled their number and booked a table for two for seven thirty. As he was making the reservation his attention was drawn to the pad beside the phone, a small notepad which had printed across the top of each page 'Kelburn Engineers' and below that the address and phone number in a plain, dark blue font.

He'd never bothered with a website because they were listed on all the online local business pages, but Bill had said a couple of times lately that they should have one to showcase what they made. After the update today Alex could see that Bill, yet again, was right, so made a mental note to look into it soon. In fact, maybe a little rethink about their letterhead, business cards and the general company image would give Alex something creative to do that was concerned with his own business.

Right now, though, he had something else to attend to. From his in-tray he took a pile of papers in different colours and sizes, letters that arrived daily at Paul's office from people who watched the show and were desperately hoping to see Alex for a personal reading. He wished he could help all these people, but there were so many it would simply be impossible, and to pick out just a few would be unfair on the rest. He always read every one of them, though, and made notes on them so a member of Paul's staff could send gentle refusals and suggestions how they could find other, equally reputable mediums to help them.

He was struggling to decipher the small, spidery handwriting of a woman who wanted to make contact with her late twin brother when his mobile rang, startling him because he was so deep in concentration. He saw that it was Paul's office and was about to answer with something sarcastic when he remembered that it wouldn't be Paul because he was still on his safari honeymoon.

"Hello?"

"Hello, Alex, it's Marcia."

Ah, Paul's very attractive, extremely efficient and rather frightening PA—until you got to know her and learnt she had a wicked sense of humour.

"Hi Marcia. How are you? I hope you're not calling with a message from my brother-in-law, because he swore to everyone that he would give one hundred per cent attention to his bride while they were on honeymoon."

"Oh, he tries calling but I just ignore him! The reason I'm ringing you is to tell you that Eselmont Productions called and they want to commission another series. Congratulations."

"Thank you! I'd expected to hear from them before now, so it's a relief to finally know. Did they say when they want filming to start?"

"They're going to get back to us with the details. They did say, though, that they want to change the format a little. They'd like for you to have an occasional guest, for instance, either to give mediumship as you do or something a little different. If you have any suggestions I can pass on to them could you email them to me? Eselmont will then check them out and see if they'll fit with what they have in mind."

Alex didn't have to think very hard about it, for one person that sprang immediately to mind was his good friend Linda Chase, a medium and healer. Linda had helped him so much after Amber had died, she deserved a shot at appearing on television, and Alex knew she'd love it and be brilliant on camera.

Two other people were also worth considering, Lars and Rosemary Magnusson, Lars was a medium, Rosemary an amazing psychic artist. They always worked together, he delivered messages and Rosemary quickly and accurately sketched in pencil or pastels those the messages were coming from.

"No problem there, Marcia, I can think of a few people straight away. Anything else?"

"Yes, a couple of other things are being considered, but they'll talk to you directly about them. One idea which seems firm, though, is one which Paul is aware of from earlier negotiations, and it's the introduction of one-to-one readings in people's own homes, so there are discussions that need to take place about the how and the who. Paul thought you should earn more now the series is such a success, so I was told to accept the commission should it come in while he was away, but to tell them that the contract is to be renegotiated on his return."

Alex thanked her again, and after asking and being told that there was nothing he needed to be doing with regard to Eselmont other than email her some names and contact details, he rang off.

The popularity of the TV series had surprised him, and it still astonished him to be recognised when he was out and about. How on earth had he leapt from working in small venues like Spiritualist churches and village halls to being a media personality with thousands clamouring to see him?

There was his autobiography too, *A Different Kind of Life*, that was, to use Paul's words, still walking off the shelves. It had humbled Alex when the book had come out and he'd travelled around doing book signings that there were so many people willing to queue for his autograph on their purchased copies.

There was more money in the bank than there'd ever been, allowing Beth to reduce her hours as an administrator at the college while she trained to become a bereavement counsellor to parents who'd lost children. It wouldn't be long, Alex thought, before she was able to work as a full-time counsellor, a job she would love and be exceptionally good at because she'd had direct experience of such loss.

Like Beth, he loved helping people. He'd been fortunate to have been born with a special gift, one he could use to bring comfort and reassurance to as many bereaved and grieving people as possible.

Television had brought him this unexpected fame,

something he was a little uncomfortable with if he was honest, but at the same time television, sensitively done, was the best way to serve very many rather than just a few. Yes, he'd be happy if he still had the time to run his engineering business himself rather than be an absent boss, but he believed that he was doing what he had been placed on this good Earth to do, and was grateful for all the hard work Paul had done on his behalf with Eselmont.

Thinking of his brother-in-law made him shake his head to remember the sequence of events that had run up to the wedding of the year. If Amber hadn't died, Beth wouldn't have insisted on a separation and Alex would not have rented the house in Saxon Road next door to Lily and Scott Miller. If he hadn't become friends with them he would never have met Lily's sister, Adele, and neither would Paul.

But he, like Maisie, could recall in clear detail Adele and Paul's first meeting, the day he and Beth, a short while after they'd reconciled, were moving out of the rented house and into their new home on the other side of town. Paul had unexpectedly turned up with Champagne (and cut crystal flutes, of course), invited himself to the farewell party at Lily's house, and Adele had been unable to take her eyes off him from the moment he'd strolled into the room as if he owned it. No-one had been surprised when the engagement had been announced just six months later.

But those happy memories brought back with a painful jolt the tragic deaths of his little girl, Amber, and of his friend Scott Miller. He needed to see Amber right now. His father had been absent a while, his attention taken up by having Alistair with him, but it was worth a try calling him, so Alex opened his mind.

"Dad. Are you there?"

He waited, but there was no response. Alex understood that his dad needed to spend time with his brother, but still he missed him responding instantly to his own need for his company. Before, he'd merely had to think of him, to call to him with his mind, and his dad had been right there in an instant.

He was caring for Amber, so any time Alex wanted to see his baby girl his dad would bring her. He was Alex's guide and gatekeeper to the spirit world, working with him every time he did a demonstration of mediumship, whether it was taking place in a village hall or the television studio, and Alex would soon need him for the new Eselmont recordings.

He called again, *"Dad?"*

But still there was no response and Alex, a little frustrated yet inwardly pleased to think of his dad and uncle having a great time together over there after so many years apart, let it go.

Beth called that she was ready, so Alex put aside thoughts of his dad and Amber and the letters that still needed to be read and set his mind to enjoying a nice meal and a bottle of good red wine with the most amazing woman in the world. The evening would end, he hoped, with a long, loving session in the metal-framed bed that he had made with his own hands as his wedding gift to her.

It had taken a while to regain the intimacy they'd enjoyed up until Amber died, but they had sensibly allowed themselves time to find their way back to each other after their reconciliation. Nowadays, Beth didn't immediately dissolve into tears after lovemaking, apologising over and over again that there could be no more children. That really didn't matter, and he was prepared to reassure her of this until his last breath. As long as he had her by his side he could cope with anything.

He grabbed his keys, rubbing the well-worn blue enamel 'A' of the keyring out of long habit. Beth was waiting for him by the front door and he gave thanks to the Universe for his great good fortune that such a wonderful, beautiful woman loved him as much as he loved her.

Chapter 8

Kallie made the usual social chit chat with the two volunteers working behind the reception desk. She then clipped the security pass to the waistband of her skirt before pushing through the double swing doors that led into the hospice wing of the huge building.

Avoiding dwelling on the entrance up ahead to the inpatients unit where her grandfather had spent his last few days, she turned right into the adjoining corridor and hesitated outside the first of the three therapy rooms. A list of available treatments was pinned on the door and she smiled to herself at the thought that this time next week she'd be administering those therapies.

Suddenly the door opened and a sandy-haired man was beaming down at her. He was dressed in a black short-sleeved tunic, black trousers and electric blue trainers. Kallie noticed he wore a copper bangle on one wrist and had an intricate Celtic band tattooed on the other.

"I had a feeling someone was out here! Not lost are you?"

"No, I'm not lost," Kallie replied, wondering how he could possibly have known she was outside the door. "I'm a holistic therapist and beautician and I'll be working here on Thursdays from next week. I'm on my way to help out in the DPU, to experience what goes on there."

The beam got wider. "Oh, it's fantastic, you'll really enjoy it. I do Thursdays as well so I guess we'll practically be roommates. I'm Kevin." He stuck out his hand and she shook it, giving her name in return. "You'll love it here, Kallie. I've been doing this for eight years and it's my favourite day of the week. We get a few coming over from the dementia wing, but it's mostly DPU guests who come to us, and if we're not too busy then any members of staff and volunteers are welcome to come and see us."

Kallie said. "I'm a little nervous about it but really looking forward to it. I'd better get a move on or I'll be late.

"Oh, that would never do!" he said with a wink. "Well, bye for now, Kallie. I look forward to seeing you around. There's no need to be nervous, you're in for a wonderful day. If you can survive the notorious induction training you can survive anything!"

Kallie laughed out loud as she waggled her fingers in farewell and walked away. Oh, that training! She had been warned that it was intense and likely to bring up all sorts of emotions, and this had turned out to be very true.

"Don't worry about crying," one of the two women giving the course had told her and the seven other new volunteers sitting in the seminar room. "Most people do get upset and it's entirely expected, so everyone's sympathetic. What happens in this room stays in this room. And we always have tissues."

This last bit made everyone break into nervous laughter as they cast sidelong glances at each other. It was a fair bet that they each had a tale of bereavement and loss to tell, and it would probably all come out over the next few sessions as they got to know each other and bonded as a group.

Kallie had found it difficult talking about the deaths of her grandparents, but she managed to get through it without too many tears. One would-be volunteer, though, had pulled out of the course after the second evening session.

They'd been shown videos of terminally-ill people talking about the different ways they were facing up to their imminent deaths. One had featured a forty-five-year-old woman who had a cardboard coffin in her living room that her children and various other members of her family were busy painting in psychedelic colours and writing messages of love to place inside. She wished to be buried in a woodland burial ground, and she had chosen the spot, written the service and made all the arrangements so her grieving family wouldn't have to. For some reason this had really upset this particular would-be volunteer and she had withdrawn. None of it had bothered Kallie as much as she'd expected, because for the most part she found everything she learned fascinating and, to her surprise, not at all depressing. In fact, it was uplifting!

This was a place where death and everything surrounding it was dealt with compassionately and without drama. They encouraged open honesty and discouraged the use of false hopes and euphemisms, telling the volunteers that it was preferable to always use straightforward language.

"We need to tell it as it is. We die. It's a fact that none of us can escape from, so let's not be embarrassed about it or skirt around the issue. Patients and their loved ones begin grieving as soon as the diagnosis is given, and this is to be expected. It's far better to be upfront and honest, and the patients you come into contact with will be grateful for it, believe me."

She had completed the training last Saturday, which had meant losing a day's earnings from the salon, and now she would lose another day by coming here to see how the DPU worked, but she considered the sacrifice more than worth it. She'd make up the money by working longer hours for a couple of months.

The DPU sitting room was empty when she entered, so she took a moment to stand in the doorway and look around to take it all in. Sofas and armchairs with brightly coloured cushions and throws scattered on them were set around three edges of the light, airy room, with a large square coffee table in the centre and side tables placed so people could put their drinks down within easy reach. Set in the far corner was a beech wood cabinet on which sat a filter coffee machine. Straight ahead of her, the top half of the wall was a single pane of glass, so the very large conservatory beyond was visible.

She could hear chatter coming from behind the closed door to her left, so she opened it carefully and found herself in a narrow kitchen where women were moving around each other as if in a well-rehearsed dance. Pam, the supervisor whom she'd met during the induction training, spotted her and called out to her.

"Welcome, Kallie. I hope you don't mind, but everyone will have to introduce themselves to you as we go along. We're one short, so your help today will be invaluable, but it means there simply isn't time to ease you in as I would've liked. Could you write your name up on the chalk board over there please? It's a Health and Safety requirement so we know which volunteers are here each day, so please remember to scrub it off before you leave. Right, let's go through to my office to get a bit of paperwork done and then you can get started."

The office turned out to be a tiny room with no windows, into which Pam had squeezed a small desk, a swivel chair on castors and a three-drawer metal filing cabinet. Kallie had to go almost up to the desk to make enough room to close the door behind her.

The two walls either side were covered in corkboards with bits of paper pinned to them and whiteboards with different coloured writing on them, and on the far wall, behind the cluttered desk, was a large holiday chart with square and round stickers all over it.

"Here's your name badge, Kallie, and this plastic folder tells you everything you need to know about setting up the DPU." She handed the items across the desk. "I know you may not be volunteering with us after this as you'll be busy giving your lovely therapies, but you might find yourself willing and able to help out now and then so do please take it home. An enterprising volunteer a couple of years back created this, taking photos to show how each area should be set up and describing how things work in the Unit. So useful for anyone new. But you'll be shown everything today, or almost everything, it does get very busy. And if you're not sure, someone will help.

"Now, most of the people who come here are receiving hospice care in their own homes, but perhaps one or two might come from the inpatient unit if they feel up to it, but all are referred to as guests, not patients. If you have any questions at any time just ask one of us, okay?"

Kallie nodded her head, taking Pam's quick glance at her wristwatch as a signal that they both needed to get out of the office and get to work helping the others get the DPU ready for that day's guests.

Pam asked her to deal with the coffee maker first. "The

instructions are on the wall behind it, and your manual will show you how things should be laid out. You'll find everything you need either in the cabinet or in the kitchen."

Following the instructions line by line, Kallie spooned the required amount of ground coffee into a new filter, added sufficient water and switched it on. She found paper napkins, plates, cups, saucers and teaspoons in the cabinet and laid them out, then, after further consulting the instruction manual, she went to the kitchen to collect the biscuit tin and a glass jar containing an assortment of wrapped sweets, making sure everything was set out so it looked just like the photograph.

Through the windows into the large conservatory, a recent add-on to give the DPU sufficient space with lots of natural light for arts and crafts, she could see Fi, a permanent member of staff she'd been introduced to during the induction training.

The short, plump woman with an untidy mass of auburn hair streaked with blue and a multitude of rings and studs in her ears and eyebrows had explained to the group all the craft activities that were available, including pottery as they'd recently installed a small kiln. Now she was setting out materials for the afternoon's session. When she glanced up and saw Kallie she gave a wave and a cheery grin, mouthing, "See you later."

Kallie wondered what kind of creative activities Fi had planned, very much looking forward to joining in.

As it was such a lovely day the conservatory was open to the gardens. Kallie could see volunteers deadheading roses and weeding flower beds, and patients and visitors sitting on benches here and there, including a man with a portable IV drip by his side who was reading a newspaper and tucking into a giant bag of crisps.

From here she had a much wider view of the extensive

gardens than the one she'd had from the small, sheltered patio of her grandad's room, and she was delighted to see the Rainstones sculpture again. She never had found the opportunity to go to the sculpture to see how the quartz sparkled and the little copper bells tinkled in the flow of water, but now she would easily be able to do so.

A woman with a tanned, heavily lined face and thick blond hair styled in a modern spiky cut, came teetering in on sky-high heels, carrying a cake on a foil-covered board.

"Kallie? Lovely to meet you. I'm Monica, practically a veteran in the DPU, and I do Tuesdays and Thursdays." She held up the cake. "This is for Bob, one of our guests. Would you be a dear and make room for it on the table, and see if you can find some candles? Oh, and matches to light them, of course. I know we have some in the kitchen somewhere. Obviously, we can't put eighty-nine candles on a cake, even if we had that many, but if you can find enough to make a good show that won't set off the sprinklers or smoke alarms that'll do."

Before Kallie managed to say a word, Monica bustled away, laughing at her own joke. She made space for the magnificent rectangular cake as asked, careful not to dip her fingers in the thick chocolate butter frosting, and found a box of candles and matches after rummaging through every drawer in the kitchen. With that mission accomplished, she was about to go in search of Pam for further instructions, when yet another volunteer came in, introduced herself, and asked Kallie to go to the dining room.

"Pam asked me to finish things in here. You'll find Trish in the dining room and she'll show you how we set up for lunch." She patted Kallie on her arm, and leaning forward and lowering her voice as if sharing a confidence, she said, "You're going to be very, very tired by the end of today."

Her head already spinning with the whirlwind of activity she was participating in, Kallie found the dining room by following the smells of hot food. Hospice inpatients had their meals in their rooms, and she'd never come here during the time her grandfather had been staying in the hospice, as she had made use of the small kitchen facilities near his room. Food and drink had been taken in the seminar room during the induction training, so she'd only seen the dining room once very briefly when they'd been given the grand tour of the whole hospice on the Saturday.

"Hello! Your badge gives you away as a volunteer, are you a newbie, Kallie?"

Kallie smiled, liking the cheerful, open expression on the woman's face. "Actually I'm a therapist. I'm going to be working in the treatment rooms on Thursdays starting next week, but I'm here to help out today so I can learn how the DPU works."

Trish indicated her own badge saying, "Mine says Patricia but everyone calls me Trish. Delighted to meet you. I'm afraid it's always a bit of a mad house before the guests arrive, but things do calm down once we're all set and everyone's settled."

"I was told how much is involved, but you really have no idea until you're part of it, do you? What would you like me to do?"

"We need to lay out our four tables over there so we can bring our guests straight in at lunch time, which is usually about half past twelve. All the other tables are for staff and visitors." Trish handed Kallie a tray of cutlery.

"We leave the chairs as they are, but be ready to whip a couple out of the way for those in wheelchairs, and offer to help anyone with sticks or walking frames. Everyone tends to want to sit in the same places every week, but Pam likes us to encourage them to move around a bit so they get to know each other better. Now, I'll pop the table cloths on and fill the water jugs, if you would please set each table with six places. That cupboard over there, the one with the dark blue doors, is ours, and that's where we keep everything: cutlery, serviettes, water glasses and wine glasses."

At Kallie's raised eyebrows, Trish said with a wide grin, "Oh yes, drinks are always on offer, provided they're not on meds that bar the consumption of alcohol, of course. We've got wine, beer and spirits, mixers, the whole works. You should have a peek in the drinks cabinet when we go back, it's pretty impressive; there are bottles of booze in there that I've never even heard of!"

The two women worked companionably together to get the tables set, and Kallie remarked how lovely it was to see how much care was taken to make it look so nice. Trish agreed, replying that she always thought the tables looked as if they belonged in a lovely little bistro, not a hospice canteen.

"Do you do any other kind of work, Trish?"

"I work in an engineering factory three days a week where they make things like iron railings and oil tanks, so it's always rather grubby, as I'm sure you can imagine. I have a tiny little office all to myself there, though, and I love the job almost as much as I love being here."

For the last task in the dining room Trish fetched two clean cotton tea towels. Handing one to Kallie, she said, "We've just got time to polish all the glasses, and let's give the cutlery a bit of a shine as well."

With less than ten minutes still to go until the Unit opened and admitted the guests, Pam called everyone together. As they gathered round Trish explained quietly to Kallie that this was an opportunity for the volunteers to sit down and draw breath while Pam went through the list of expected guests, giving brief outlines of their illnesses and current treatments. Kallie saw Kevin with another tunic-wearing therapist and waved.

Pam addressed Kallie. "You'll be working in the therapy rooms after today, but it's worthwhile for you to come and listen to this bit if you can so you'll know in advance what's going on medically with anyone who comes from here to you for a treatment. If you are asked to give a treatment to anyone from the dementia wing you'll be told what you need to know by whoever brings them over."

Pam ended by telling them of one recent death, all in the matter of fact manner that was the way of the hospice. At last all was ready, and the guests started to arrive, brought by friends, family members or volunteer drivers. There was a flurry of activity as everyone was welcomed into the room and seated. The volunteers organised coffees and teas and passed round the tin of biscuits, and when everyone was settled and comfortable Pam asked that all the volunteers sit down again so she could begin.

"Let's get the sad news over with first," she said. "I'm sorry to tell you that Alfred died on Monday. He was at home with his family, and it was very peaceful. I don't yet know the funeral arrangements, but as soon as we hear I'll let those of you who wish to go know when and where it's to be."

Pam paused to let the news sink in, and Kallie felt the atmosphere in the room sink a little. This was a necessary announcement, she supposed, otherwise people would notice that a guest was missing and would be wondering and asking where they were. It was right and proper that Pam tell them straight away, for this was a hospice and anyone attending the DPU knew that their own deaths would likely occur within months, a year, or maybe two years at the most.

Pam rustled the papers on her lap and, with a much lighter, happier voice, she gestured first to a young woman in a wheelchair then to Kallie herself. "I'd like you all to welcome new guest Louise, and also Kallie Harper, who will be starting next week as a therapist. She'll be here every Thursday, so if you'd like a treatment from her there are leaflets on the coffee table listing everything she offers, which includes massage, Reiki healing and aromatherapy. Kevin and Chris are here today, so just let someone know if you want to see them and we'll get you booked in."

There were murmurs of appreciation, and Kallie heard a woman, whose head was wrapped in a colourful scarf, say to the person sitting next to her that she would love a head massage because her hair was growing back and her scalp itched.

Pam waited a moment, then said, "And finally, let's all wish our Bob over there a very happy birthday! We'll have the lovely cake his niece made after lunch, so do please leave a little room for it."

After a few more items of news covering general hospice matters, including a night-time fundraising half-marathon that Kallie thought she might like to sign up for, it was time to top up the hot and cold drinks, offer more biscuits, go round with the lunch menu and take orders and, when all that was done, sit and chat with the guests. She headed for Bob, opening the conversation by asking about his birthday plans.

He chuckled and replied, "I think the family will insist on taking me out to dinner tonight, though I don't have much of an appetite these days and am happy with scrambled egg and bacon. I thought I'd be gone by now because of the damned cancer eating away at my insides and here I am at eighty-nine and still breathing. Ridiculous."

Liking the twinkle in the old man's eyes, Kallie said, "Why is it ridiculous, Bob? It's quite an achievement, surely?"

He was a tiny man, almost swallowed up by the high-backed armchair he was sitting in. His grin showing a row of crooked teeth with a front one missing, Bob nodded towards the cake and said, with a broad Wiltshire accent, "Tell you what'll be an achievement, and that's if I can blow out them candles without needing to be resuscitated and then eat any of the cake without getting most of it down the front of my shirt."

Kallie sat with him for five more minutes, enjoying the warmth and charm, the sparky humour he displayed. Bob was entertaining and funny and she would have liked to stay with him, to hear his whole life story, but he tapped her on the knee and said, "You'd best work the room a little, love, or I'll be accused of monopolising the prettiest volunteer in the place. Go on, now, someone else'll soon be over to keep me company."

Giving him a playful tap on his arm for his delightful compliment, which she was sure he used on all the ladies, Kallie glanced around to see where to go next. Her eyes alighted on the new guest, Louise, but Trish was sitting with her and didn't look like she was going to move on to someone else. Louise had the most beautiful hair, dark brown with coppery streaks, thick and wavy, and so long it spilled down the back of the wheelchair almost to the seat. Trish was chatting to her quietly, and Kallie thought back over what Pam had said about Louise's condition. The young woman was unable to talk, yet Kallie could see that Trish was giving her every ounce of focus and attention, as if she was having the most riveting conversation ever.

As if sensing she was being watched, Trish glanced up and smiled warm encouragement to Kallie before offering Louise a plastic beaker with a straw in it. Kallie decided to go over to a very handsome man who she thought might be in his early forties, who had the deepest blue eyes she had ever seen.

When he introduced himself Kallie recalled Pam saying that he had an inoperable brain tumour. During training, she'd been told not to talk about their illnesses unless they mentioned it first, but to concentrate instead on who they were and everyday things they liked to try and keep things light and cheerful. She asked John if he liked to join in with the afternoon arts and crafts sessions, and he told her he had trouble with his co-ordination and preferred to stay in the lounge, but sometimes he brought his guitar and played for everyone.

"For some reason I can still play well," he said. "I used to be able to sing pretty well, too, but nowadays I can't hold the tune and I forget the words. I miss singing almost more than anything else."

The smile never left his face as he answered Kallie's questions about his music and his family, and everything was explained to her without any self-pity or anger, just a matter-of-factness that she really admired.

At half past twelve it was time to take everyone to lunch, so Trish took Kallie under her wing again as they helped move guests to the cafeteria. Pam indicated which table the volunteers should sit at, and Kallie had to admit to herself that she was relieved none of the guests in her care would need her help with eating or drinking. She was quite capable of doing it, but these people didn't know her and she wouldn't be with them next week, so it seemed best to let the regular volunteers undertake such an intimate task.

Trish stayed with Louise, as they had already formed a bond during the morning. It was a lovely, congenial forty-five minutes, with good conversation and lots of laughter, and then it was time to go back to the Unit and everyone except John went straight into the conservatory to spend a couple of hours being creative with Fi.

About halfway through the afternoon, the birthday cake was served with more hot drinks and after that it seemed no time at all before the guests had gone and the DPU had been set back in order for the following day. Kallie used the blackboard eraser to rub out her name and was on her way back to reception to sign out of the visitors' book when Trish caught up with her.

"How are you after your baptism of fire in the DPU?"

Kallie laughed. "Absolutely exhausted but deeply satisfied with myself. I woke up in the early hours feeling really nervous, and I honestly wondered if I'd be up to it, but I loved every minute of it. Everyone's so positive, aren't they? Amazing people, all of them. I'm so looking forward to being in the therapy room next week, today really helped me prepare for it."

"I'm glad you feel that way. This is such a happy place, which comes as a major surprise to many, let me tell you! But, as you probably found out, not everyone makes it through the training course, and the reality of working or volunteering here can prove too much for some. Most of us volunteers come here because we've had family members looked after here. In my case it was my older half-sister. Motor neurone disease, like Louise. She got her wish to die here, because she loved the gardens so."

"I'm so sorry, it's a dreadful disease," Kallie said. "My grandfather died here too. His body was simply worn out with old age, and his passing was very peaceful. When I discovered the therapy rooms on one of my visits I knew I wanted to work here. I love the salon where I work, it's a pretty building in the most beautiful country setting, and now I've got Thursdays to look forward to in this fabulous place as well."

Trish regarded Kallie with steady, light brown eyes. "Patients really appreciate the treatments you give, especially things like aromatherapy. Even acupuncture is popular; I've never tried it but I'm told you really can't feel the needles. They're so used to painful injections and blood tests and pills and all the other not-so-pleasant stuff they have to endure, that spending time with someone like you is just the tonic they need." Her eyes sparkled as she said, "Did they tell you that volunteers can have treatments as well? If you do hot stones massages I'll be forever your friend."

"Are you parked outside?" asked Kallie. "My car's way over in front of the dementia wing."

"In that case you may as well walk with me through the building and go out through the dementia wing exit. I'm going to sit with my dad for an hour." At the look of surprise on Kallie's face, she explained, "Oh, sorry, I hadn't mentioned that, had I? Here's another shocker for you, my dad's a hundred years old and fast heading to being one of the oldest surviving dementia patients."

She explained to Kallie that her father had been married three times and that she, his youngest, had been born when he was in his sixties. "My mum looked after him for as long as she could, but she's thirty years younger and it didn't seem fair to keep her tied to someone who no longer even recognised her. Mum adored him and he was the best of dads; the diagnosis hit us all hard, but especially her. I'm happy to say, though, that she has found happiness with a new partner who we all love. I'm the only one of the family still local so I sit with him just about every day. Come on, I'll show you the way; it's safer than weaving your way through that car park at this time of day when so many cars are coming and going."

Kallie confided as they walked along that she didn't know who her father was, and her mother had been nearly forty when she had her. "So that makes us both the product of an older parent, though I'm an only child. I suppose being raised by your dad was a bit like me being brought up by my grandparents? Age means nothing, though, does it? It's all about how young we are inside."

Feeling she had made a new friend, Kallie said goodbye to Trish and went wearily to her car. By the time she got home she was so tired she fell asleep on the sofa for an hour, only waking up because she was hungry and thirsty.

Chapter 9

Sylvia peered into the cupboard under the stairs but couldn't see what she was looking for. She reached round for the pull cord to turn on the light and then saw that what she wanted was right at the back, just visible behind the vacuum cleaner, ironing board, laundry basket and sewing machine. Tutting at the thought of hauling everything out, she heard Simon's cheerful whistling as he came in from the garden.

"Could you get the clock down for me please so I can change the battery? I can't get to the step stool without emptying the cupboard."

He reached up and took off its hook. "I'll see to it."

"Okay, I'll get a new ba . . ."

But he had turned away from her, whistling a different tune, heading for his workshop with the clock tucked under his arm.

Deciding to leave him to it, even though it meant it probably wouldn't be put back on the wall for several hours because he always got distracted by something else he was working on, Sylvia went outside to deadhead some roses.

As she ambled amongst the flower beds, she couldn't help but think about the increasingly worrying symptoms Simon was showing. His anxiety over whether he had his wallet and that the doors were locked every time they went out, or up to bed, didn't cause her too much alarm, but the tantrum over the wedding outfit had been shocking. Then he'd left the hat behind at the reception and seemed to have entirely forgotten that the suit was on hire and needed to be returned.

His changeable moods were making things increasingly difficult, with Sylvia constantly having to soothe and placate him, even though she didn't know half the time what had upset him.

The old Simon would apologise and immediately try to make amends, but this Simon sometimes looked at her with pure dislike, and that was like a knife being thrust into her heart. Would he go to the doctor if she asked him?

She paused at the sight of a particularly beautiful rose with perfect petals, creamy yellow with a golden centre, and bent to smell its soft perfume, asking herself why she was hesitating to talk to him about this. They talked about everything, every little thing, it was the basis of the enduring strength of their long marriage, but she was so worried about what the episodes of forgetfulness and bad temper might mean she couldn't bring herself to voice her concerns out loud.

She wasn't even sure if Simon was aware of his changed behaviour. How would she even raise the subject? "Hey, husband, do you know what a pain you've become lately? Do you think you might have Alzheimer's?" Even thinking the 'A' word made her shudder, she couldn't possibly suggest to Simon that he might have it.

But what if it were the other way round? She sat back on her heels and looked up at the sky. What if it was her manner that was changing in a worrying way, if it was her forgetting things and fretting over inconsequential stuff all the time, wouldn't she want Simon to tell her? She was sure she would, and she was also sure that she would make an appointment with her doctor straight away and deal with it.

"Tonight," she told herself. "I'll tackle it tonight."

An hour later she went inside to make lunch. There was still no clock on the wall and no sign of Simon, so she got a new battery and went to his workshop. On the workbench, lined up neatly in a row, were the clock components of back plate, clear plastic front, black metal hands, movement mechanism, screws and battery casing. The dead battery had been placed in a chipped glass ashtray that Simon kept despite giving up smoking decades ago.

Simon had his back to her, rummaging through a drawer. When he turned around he was holding a tiny screwdriver and a magnifying glass.

With a teasing note in her voice, she pointed and asked, "Did you take it apart deliberately or did you accidentally drop it?"

"What do you mean? Of course I didn't drop it."

"But why is it in pieces? It only nee . . ."

Looking annoyed, he interrupted her and spoke with exasperation, "You know why! It stopped working. You asked me to fix it and I'm fixing it!"

Feeling that horrible prickle of unease at the tone of his voice and the expression in his eyes she stared back at him, knowing he wasn't joking but nevertheless wishing passionately that he was.

"It stopped working because it needs a new battery, love, that's all." She held out the one she had in her hand.

Simon's mouth worked as he looked from Sylvia to all the

bits on the bench, and she willed him to laugh, to tell her that he just wanted to see how it worked and have the challenge of putting the clock back together again, even though that in itself would be unusual. He could put up curtain poles and hang pictures so they were straight, he could make bird boxes out of bits of wood, screws and nails, but he was hopeless at fixing anything with moving parts.

Placing the new battery beside the pieces of the clock, Sylvia suggested he come in for lunch, and turned to lead the way out. But, two steps away from the workshop, she heard Simon curse and turned in time to witness him sweep everything off the bench with his arm.

Bits of plastic and metal hit the wooden floor and bounced and rolled, the smallest screws falling straight through a hole in the floor, but Simon didn't stop to pick them up. He marched out, pushing roughly past Sylvia, and stalked away across the garden and into the street.

Shocked and fighting back tears, Sylvia watched him go, deciding not to chase after him. She wouldn't talk to him about her worries when he came back either. He'd need time to calm down, she needed time to work out exactly what to say and how to say it.

I can't do it today, she thought. *I'll wait a bit longer, until I know it's the right time.*

When an hour had passed with no sign of Simon returning, Sylvia ate her lunch and left a covered plate of ham salad sandwiches for when he came back. Maybe he'd gone to the pub and had a bite to eat there, or maybe he was just walking off his temper.

As time ticked on with no sign of his return she found herself changing her mind yet again, concluding that she simply must initiate a discussion with him when he got back. For too long she'd been flip-flopping like this over whether to talk to him or not, but the manner of his disappearance today combined with the realisation that there would never be a 'right' time finally brought matters to a head. She had no choice now but to tackle him head on so they could do something about it.

He was brought home three hours later by their next-door neighbour, Len Keene, who looked very worried. He had Simon by the elbow on one side and his well-behaved, graceful dark grey lurcher on the other. The dog sat patiently outside as Len led Simon into the house.

"I was walking past the pub and I saw him sitting at one of the tables outside, just staring into space. I spoke to him, asked him if he wanted to come inside and have a pint with me, but . . . well, it was as if he didn't know me. Didn't seem to know where he was, either, so I brought him back. Is everything all right, love? He hasn't had a knock on the head or anything, has he?"

Hiding how frantic she had become during the long wait and swallowing down the tears of anger and relief that threatened now he was safely returned, Sylvia managed a bright smile and told Len an outright lie. "He's on a new medication for high blood pressure and it seems not to be agreeing with him. You know, sleepless nights, a bit of confusion, that kind of thing. It needs to be changed again, obviously. Thank you so much, Len, for bringing him home."

Len seemed happy to accept her explanation. Sylvia, out of politeness, offered tea and was relieved when Len refused, saying that it was the dog's dinner time. He left to go next door and no doubt tell his wife all about Simon's strange episode.

She sat Simon down in the living room and pulled the foot

stool over so she could sit directly in front of him. Their knees touching, she took both his hands in hers and shook them gently.

"Simon? Can you hear me?"

Apparently, he could not, or if he could, he was ignoring her or was incapable of responding. Pushing away a flutter of fear, Sylvia rose and went to the phone, scrolling quickly to the number of their doctor's surgery. She explained to the receptionist what had happened, and was told to bring Simon over in an hour, if she could. Their own doctor was not available to see them, but they had an emergency appointment available with someone else if she was happy to see him instead.

Twenty minutes after their appointed time they were sitting in front of Dr Marsden, a much younger man than their usual doctor.

Simon was becoming more responsive but was still a bit dazed. Sylvia quickly explained everything that had been happening, and what had happened that morning. Dr Marsden asked lots of questions about Simon's age and if he had been in an accident where he'd hit his head, if he'd complained of headaches, and if there were any medical issues Sylvia thought could be relevant.

Thinking of how she'd lied to Len Keene, she shook her head, saying that her husband didn't even have any of the usual things associated with age, such as high blood pressure, high cholesterol, blood sugar issues, hearing loss. Not even arthritis in any joints. She spoke the dreaded words, the first time she'd said them out loud: "I'm worried that it's Alzheimer's."

Looking sympathetic, Dr Marsden told her not to jump to conclusions. "We need to do some tests, including a brain scan, so I'll make the appointments." he said. "Diagnosis takes time, though, and isn't always definitive when it comes to dementia, so I can't offer any treatment until we know what it is we're dealing with. In the meantime, I can only suggest you keep a close eye on him and make sure he comes to no harm. Have you family nearby? Close friends?"

When she said yes to both, he continued, "Then I suggest you let them know what's happening so they can help you. I appreciate you may want to keep things to yourself until you know for sure what's going on, but it wouldn't be wise to try and cope with it on your own."

He talked some more about the possibilities of what might be ailing Simon, including minor stroke or brain tumour, and advised her to pick up some leaflets from reception on her way out so she and her family could read about the symptoms to look out for.

As he finished speaking, Simon suddenly snapped out of his trance and demanded to know where he was. When Sylvia told him, worried that he would get angry again, Simon simply said, "Oh" and meekly allowed the doctor to ask him some questions, check his blood pressure, examine his eyes and ears and take a blood test.

They left the doctor's office with the promise that they would be contacted soon about the brain scan and other tests, and Sylvia decided not to pick up any leaflets yet as she didn't want Simon seeing them. There was no point scaring themselves unnecessarily. Wait until they knew.

In the car, Simon hesitated as he pulled the seatbelt round himself and asked who needed a brain scan and why. Trying not to cry Sylvia said they needed to get home so they could talk face to face, relieved when Simon didn't demand to have the conversation there and then. She drove home with her mind whirring.

It was obvious to her that something was very wrong with Simon, whether it be a stroke, tumour, neither of which she'd considered until the doctor mentioned it, or Alzheimer's. Which would be preferable, she wondered: a tumour that could possibly be operated on, or dementia, which had no cure? She knew she needed to tell Anna, Paul and Beth about what was happening, but not today. She'd been indecisive for too long about Simon and didn't want to make the same mistake again, but she couldn't take any more today. She would wait until they had a firm diagnosis and tell the family immediately. Right now, all she wanted to do was get home with Simon and lock all the doors.

Chapter 10

Averting her eyes from the things that had been her gran's favourites and wondering if she'd ever forget the small details, Kallie briskly pushed the trolley up and down the supermarket aisles.

After Walter had died she'd struggled to get used to shopping for just her and Gran, but then Verity had passed away within months of Walter and even now Kallie did not enjoy shopping for one. Putting a packet of pasta next to the potatoes, chocolates, sweets and peanuts already in the basket, she headed for the dairy section.

A man about her age, medium height and good looking, an empty basket on his arm, was browsing the shelves and when she selected the butter she wanted he asked her if it was good for frying with. For a brief moment she wondered if it was a chat-up line, but he didn't even look at her face; he genuinely wanted her opinion on the attributes of a particular brand of butter and that was all.

Suddenly depressed, for here she was, not yet thirty and no romance since the love of her life had announced that she was not the love of his life, Kallie ignored the low-fat yogurt she had been intending to buy and headed for the freezer section. She selected a large tub of salted caramel ice cream, hoping that it might, just might, make her feel better. She chose the self-checkout to pay for her purchases, glad that for once she got everything through without a hitch, and left for home.

When she pulled up in front of the tiny cottage that had been her home since she'd been born, she switched off the engine and stared at the white-painted house that she adored. But would she ever get used to this; coming home to an empty, silent place? Verity had always made sure Walter and Kallie were given a good welcome home, the gentle tones of Classical FM or BBC Radio 4 playing in the background, the delicious smells of their supper wafting from the kitchen. They would eat together at the kitchen table, crammed between the fridge freezer and the back door, Verity wanting to hear all about their day.

After Walter's death her gran had tried to keep things going as normal for her and Kallie, but in her last few weeks Kallie had not had a welcome home when she got in from work for lunch or at the end of the day, finding instead that Verity had spent most of the time sleeping.

With a deep sigh, she grabbed the shopping and her handbag and marched up the short path and through the door, stepping straight into the living room. Kicking aside the local paper and the post lying on the mat, most of it probably junk mail, Kallie carried her purchases to the kitchen and put everything away.

Checking the kettle had sufficient water, she switched it on then changed her mind and poured a glass of cold white wine instead. Holding the glass by its stem, she stared out into the garden, a small square patch of lawn edged with flower beds in serious need of attention. Her gran had mostly tended the garden, with Kallie joining her sometimes at the weekends to potter rather uselessly about, but she hadn't had the heart to do more than mow the grass and pull a few weeds since Verity had died. She must get out there soon. She didn't have the gardening skills to return it to its former glory, but she was determined to try both for her own satisfaction and to honour the memory of her grandparents.

The phone rang and she dashed back into the living room to grab it before the answering machine switched on, wondering if it would be her mother. Celia was the only one who used the landline, all her friends and clients called Kallie on her mobile.

"Hello?"

Instead of her mother's clipped greeting there was nothing but crackling on the line, and she waited for Celia or someone else to speak. Nothing. She placed the receiver back on the cradle, noticing for the first time the blinking red light. There were six new messages. Six! She pressed the button, listening to them one by one just long enough to know there was nothing but the crackling sound, and then she deleted them, cursing all call centres for that was surely what was going on here.

Just as she deleted the last one her mobile trilled and seeing that it was Rosa, she answered it with a cheerful hello, grinning as her best friend greeted her in her usual singsong way, "Hi Kallie! What are you up to?"

"Well, I was planning on spending my evening with a tub of salted caramel ice cream and a glass of wine, unless you have a better offer?"

Rosa laughed. "Not for tonight, dear heart, but are you doing anything tomorrow? Mark's working late and I've got it into my head to go to the cinema and then have a bite to eat, but I don't want to go by myself. You up for it?"

"Great idea. What are we going to see?"

Rosa told her the choices and they settled on a film and a time to meet. Immensely cheered, Kallie decided she didn't need the comfort of ice cream after all and wondered whether, as she was in such a good mood thanks to her ever-cheerful friend, she ought to call her mother, ought being the operative word, because they were no more than duty calls and she found her mother very hard to talk to. She hadn't seen Celia face to face since the day of Verity's funeral, when they had rowed, as usual, and her mother had flounced out in a huff.

For the millionth time, Kallie thought to herself, *Why, oh why, can we not be in the same room for longer than five minutes without arguing?*

She took a large slug of wine because there was no answer to that question but now her head was filled with unwelcome reflections on her difficult mother. The old carriage clock on the mantelpiece chimed the hour, bringing Kallie out of trying to decipher her difficult relationship with her mother, and she decided not to make the call, for her good mood had somewhat dissipated and talking to Celia would only make it worse.

She took a long, hot soak in the bath, perfumed with some of her special oils to lift her spirits, then made some supper and placed it on a lap tray so she could eat while watching television. She was halfway through a sitcom that actually made her laugh out loud when the channel suddenly changed. Surprised, Kallie wondered if she was sitting on the remote but, no, there it was on the cushion beside her.

Putting the lap tray and her half-eaten dinner on the floor, she picked up the remote, shook it, and pressed the buttons hard in an effort to get back to the channel she had been watching. As if it had developed a mind of its own, the TV switched back and forth between the channel she wanted to watch and one showing a documentary about deep sea fishing that she wasn't the least bit interested in. Thoroughly exasperated she pressed the off button on the remote and the screen went blank.

"Oh, so you'll turn off but you won't let me watch my programme? I can't afford to replace you, you know!" she said to the empty room.

There was a faint click and the television came back on to the right channel.

Bemused, Kallie picked up her supper again. "It's just an electrical glitch," she muttered under her breath. "Just like the lights. This old place probably needs rewiring."

For a couple of weeks the landing light had been switching on and off by itself, and now with the TV playing up as well, she knew she would have to get an electrician in, and hoped it wouldn't cost too much.

The television behaved itself for the rest of the evening and she was able to finish her meal uninterrupted and watch the programmes she wanted to see. When the ten o'clock news ended she started to carry the lap tray and her empty plate through to the kitchen to wash up, but the landing light came on, stopping her in her tracks.

It hadn't bothered her when this particular glitch had manifested not long ago, but this time the hairs on her arms had raised because it felt as if she was standing in a field of static. It spooked her, and made her wonder anew about the occasions when things had gone missing that she'd put down to her absent mindedness. How many times had she put things down and when she went to pick them up later they weren't there? When she eventually found the item it was always somewhere she could have put them, but knew she hadn't.

This is what had happened with her car keys this morning. She'd been ready to go to work and had automatically reached into the dish, the one she'd made years ago at school, and the keys hadn't been there. She'd stared down at the crudely painted pattern on the bottom of the empty dish for a full ten seconds, not believing her own eyes. She had thrown the keys in that dish when she had come in from work yesterday, just as she always did. But they weren't there, so the only conclusion she could come to was that she must have put them down somewhere else.

She went from room to room searching, then, when she didn't find them, replayed in her mind her return home, picturing herself coming through the door with the keys in her hand. There'd been no post on the mat, no flashing light on the answering machine. She had switched on the television as she always did, just to fill the empty house with sound. She knew she had placed the keys in the pot.

She really needed to be on her way to work or risk being late for her first client, but she searched everywhere again, including pockets, drawers and under the furniture. She'd tipped the contents of her handbag onto the floor and put everything back item by item.

No keys.

Baffled and feeling quite exasperated with herself, she'd gone to get a glass of water, and there they were, by the sink. Unable to explain it other than a complete memory lapse, she'd just grabbed them and run out of the house.

When she'd come home again, she had very carefully and very consciously, placed the keys in the dish, listening to them clink as they settled against the fired clay. Throughout the evening her eyes had been drawn to them, and she looked at them now, the end of her car key poking just above the rim of the dish. What if she were to wash up her dishes, come back in, and find they weren't there?

Feeling silly and self-conscious, yet compelled to speak out loud, she said, "Grandad? Gran? Are you two playing games with me?"

She had never given any serious thought to the possibility of communication with loved ones who had passed away, but her grandmother had constantly claimed that Walter was with her in those last months she was alive. He was keeping them company, she'd insisted, and Kallie hadn't questioned it or contradicted her because it had cheered Verity immensely to think he was always around, and it cheered Kallie too.

Thinking about it now, though, she wondered if both of them really could be watching over her and rather welcomed the idea of it even if she couldn't really believe it. Many other holistic therapists she knew believed fervently in life after death and fairies and the power of crystals and angels . . . Oh, there was quite a list. Kallie herself admitted that she simply wasn't sure about such things.

When she'd been a little girl, Walter had made up stories to scare her about the cottage being haunted because of its great age and its proximity to the thirteenth century church and its graveyard.

But when she'd stared wide-eyed at him, her little body beginning to tremble, he'd taken her in his arms and told her that there were no such things as ghosts and she had nothing to be afraid of, ever. He explained that the noises she heard in the dead of night were nothing but the skittering and scratching of little furry mice in the thatch and the old floorboards creaked because of changes in temperature. These were normal things that one expected in a place that was hundreds of years old. Walter had always made her feel safe.

"I'd love it if it is you two trying to make your presence known, but I'm going to need a little more convincing please!"

She stood stock still at the bottom of the stairs, clutching the lap tray, her ears straining to hear anything, eyes alert in case anything moved. But nothing happened. She left the landing light on and carried on into the kitchen.

With her hands in the washing up bowl cleaning her plate and cutlery, she almost jumped out of her skin when the TV volume suddenly blared, so painfully loud it caused her to yelp in surprise. She ran in, hands dripping, and turned it down, but now she was rattled, and suddenly her fear changed to overwhelming grief for her grandparents and she started to cry.

The landline started ringing again and though she was tempted to let it go through to the answering machine she scrubbed her tears away and answered it. All she heard was a crackling sound.

Chapter 11

"I feel weird."

Simon looked up from his newspaper, peering over his reading glasses to where Sylvia was sitting across from him, and was alarmed to see how white her face was. Most people would say they felt ill, or unwell, or a little off colour, but not his Sylvia.

"What do you mean by weird?"

"It's hard to explain, but I didn't sleep well and I haven't felt right since I woke up, to be honest. I thought it was indigestion, but I've never had it like this. Whatever it is, it's getting worse by the minute."

He crossed the room to her, brushing her fringe back to feel her forehead. She wasn't hot, but her skin felt clammy. "A cold coming on, d'you think?"

Sylvia frowned as she rubbed her jaw. "More like flu. We should have had those jabs. You'd better go and get one as soon as possible, love, we can't risk both of us being ill!"

In all the years since reaching eligibility for the annual flu vaccination, they had joined the long queues at the local health centre. But this time, after long discussions about the benefits versus the side effects and the possibility that the media reports were correct that they hadn't got the formula right, Sylvia had made a convincing argument for not going ahead. The letter informing them of the date of this year's vaccination at their local surgery had gone straight into the bin and he'd thought no more about it. But, as she said, they ought to have the vaccination if it was still possible to do so.

"Okay, I'll sort it out. But what can I do for you now? Would you like a cup of tea? Aspirin?"

Sylvia shook her head, still rubbing her jaw. "I'm sorry, Simon, but I feel a bit sick. Could you get me a bowl from the kitchen? I don't know if I'm going to be, but I know I wouldn't be able to make it to the bathroom in time."

Worried, for Sylvia had never been like this in all the years they'd been married, he hurried off and opened and closed cupboard doors in frustration, staring like an idiot at the immaculately ordered shelves, not seeing anything but cups, mugs and small glass dessert dishes. Then he caught sight of the washing-up bowl in the sink, glad that it was empty and clean, and grabbed that. By the time he got back to Sylvia, her face had changed from white to ash grey and she was hugging herself, arms across her chest, hands gripping her shoulders so her knuckles were white. She rocked herself backwards and forwards.

"Sylvia? Hey, sweetheart, you're scaring me now. Tell me how you feel. Where exactly does it hurt?"

Sweat beaded on her upper lip as through clenched teeth she managed to say, "Everywhere. Call the doctor," before she burst into tears.

"Sod that, I'm calling an ambulance!"

Keeping his eyes fixed on Sylvia as he dialled 999 and talked to the emergency services operator, he gave their address, her name, her age, stumbling over a couple of the details. He described her symptoms, trying to keep the wobble out of his voice as he looked at his beloved wife across the room from him, suffering and in pain.

He was assured that an ambulance was already on its way and he should stay on the line until the paramedics arrived.

"Hurry up!" Simon shouted and he hardly heard the soothing voice of the operator telling him to keep calm, asking questions about Sylvia that he couldn't answer because his brain felt like it was melting inside his skull.

Everything then went simultaneously super-fast and super-slow in a confusion of action and noise. When Sylvia slumped to the floor onto her knees, he hardly heard the despatcher telling him to open the front door for the medics to get in as soon as they arrived because he dropped the handset and rushed over to her.

He could hear the siren getting louder as it neared the house. Telling Sylvia that help had arrived, he tried to hold her up but she fought him, wanting to stay lying down. Then there was the ringing of the doorbell and a pounding of the knocker, and he forced himself to leave her and let them in.

The room abruptly seemed full of people, though there were only two male medics; one in his fifties, Simon guessed, the other quite a bit younger and so broad-shouldered and muscular it was a wonder they found a uniform to fit him. The older man went straight to Sylvia, talking in a low, soft voice that seemed to reassure her, the other one addressed Simon.

He indicated the handset on the floor by the table. "May I tell the despatcher that we're here, sir?"

"Oh, yes, yes, of course. I'm sorry. I . . ."

The medic put a reassuring hand on Simon's arm. "Don't you worry about it, sir."

He spoke into the phone and replaced it on its cradle before joining his colleague, the pair of them talking in low voices to Sylvia and conferring between themselves.

Simon knew that he had to let them get on with it but it was hard to just stand there doing nothing while they helped Sylvia to lay out flat on the carpet and took her pulse and blood pressure. Simon became aware of a portable ECG machine on the floor by Sylvia's side, a display of lines dancing across the small screen in time to Sylvia's heart rhythms. He was aware too of Sylvia being asked questions, and questions being asked of him. He knew he should answer them, but he couldn't find his voice. He was frozen, just wishing the whole terrifying scene wasn't happening.

But if it had to happen, why not to him? Why should it be his Sylvia who suffered this way? Could it be, as she suspected, a severe case of flu?

Flu killed people, he knew that, especially older people, and he cursed himself for acquiescing to Sylvia's decision not to have the vaccinations. And they were old, he realised with a jolt. Okay, he knew he had memory lapses, but that was normal at his time of life. He and Sylvia ensured that they kept active, mentally and physically, and they had a wonderful social life, hobbies that they did individually or together, lots of trips around the country and abroad. They were planning a cruise to see the Northern Lights.

The younger paramedic was talking to him again, and although Simon understood what he was being told, the man's voice sounded as if it came from a long way away. The ECG readings showed that Sylvia was having a problem, the medic explained, and the mask over her face was to give her a little extra oxygen.

They lifted her onto a wheeled stretcher that Simon had no recollection of being brought in. They were going to take her to hospital. They were asking did he want to go in the ambulance with them or follow in his own car. Of course, he wanted to go with them. He wasn't going to let her out of his sight.

As he followed them outside, having the presence of mind to put on a jacket, pick up his keys, wallet and mobile phone from the hall table, it started to feel as if he were wading through treacle. And their voices, the medics' voices, he could no longer make out their words.

Their next-door neighbour was at the gate, a kind woman they'd known for years yet he simply could not recall her name. He could see her mouth moving, but it was as if his ears were stuffed with cotton wool and he could not understand her. He registered the concern on her face, though, even managed a weak smile to acknowledge it, as he climbed into the back of the ambulance like a robot and sat where he was told to.

"I have to go back, I've forgotten my wallet."

"I'm sorry sir, but we really can't delay."

About to object, Simon searched his pockets, relieved to feel the wallet and keys there. He steadied himself as the ambulance set off, lights flashing and siren wailing.

After that it was as if he'd passed into another dimension, one where he had no control, no part to play, no say in anything that was happening.

Within moments of arriving at the hospital Sylvia's stretcher disappeared and he had been politely but firmly held back by a male nurse, forced to answer yet more questions. But he had to, for her sake. Again, as with the emergency services operator, he recited her full name and her age. He gave her date of birth. Told the nurse making the notes she'd always been healthy, seldom got a cold, never complained of headaches. She suffered from hay fever every May.

When a doctor came out and informed him Sylvia was having a heart attack and that she needed emergency bypass surgery he didn't believe it and started to shout at him. The doctor remained calm, compassion in his eyes, until Simon ran out of rant and stood there, wide-eyed, panting and terrified.

"Is there anyone you'd like us to call, Mr Savarese? A family member perhaps who could come and wait with you?"

It was then, finally, he realised how serious the situation was and he would have to contact Anna with this awful news.

"It's okay, thank you. I'll call my daughter." He pulled the mobile phone from his pocket.

"You can't use that in here, I'm afraid. Just go outside a little way and it'll be fine."

With a shaking hand, he started to search for Anna's number, but the names on the tiny screen were blurred and he pressed the wrong one. He hung up and tried again, but his mind went blank and he couldn't think of the name he was searching for. He stared in panic as he scrolled through the list, his mouth going dry, because now he had no idea where he was and who he was meant to be calling.

Frantic, he darted back through the automatic doors into A&E, saw people on rows of chairs, sitting motionless and blank-eyed, or sipping coffee, or idly chatting. Staff members dressed in trousers and tunics in different shades of green, burgundy and blue, some with stethoscopes round their necks or poking out of large pockets, some with upside down watches pinned on the tunics, were coming and going. He took in all this detail, yet couldn't remember what he was doing there.

Then, just as the receptionist called out to him, a concerned expression on her face, that moment of feeling utterly lost passed as quickly as it had come, and he dashed outside, found his daughter's phone number, which was, of course, at the top of the list, and called it before he could forget again.

She answered with such a cheerful hello that he choked up and could barely get the words out to tell her what had happened. Before he finished speaking Anna was crying, but she told him she was on her way, and the phone went dead.

Simon didn't know how long he waited, but at last there she was, rushing into the A&E waiting room, her frantic eyes searching him out. Close behind her came Beth and Alex, and Simon thanked them for bringing her, remembering that his son-in-law, Felix, was away on a business trip.

Alex shook Simon's outstretched hand and asked what was happening. Simon could only swing his head from side to side and tell them that Sylvia had had a heart attack and been rushed into surgery.

"I'll go and see if I can find out anything more," Alex said, and walked over to the reception desk.

Simon hugged his daughter close, then drew Beth to him as well, fighting back tears as he offered his handkerchief to Anna. Eventually, she sniffed and pulled away so she could look at him.

"A heart attack, Dad? I can't believe it."

"Nor me, Anna, my love. Nor me."

Beth asked what had happened, but before he could answer Alex came back over to them. "They can't, or won't, tell me anything more than you already know, Simon. Sylvia's going to be in surgery for a couple of hours, though, maybe more, so they suggest we go to the cafeteria and have a hot drink, try to eat something, because it'll be a long while before you can see her."

Anna, highly distressed, said that they should stay where they were, but Alex, pointing out that there did not seem to be enough seats for them to sit together, convinced her that they should do as suggested and go to the café.

"They won't bring her back here anyway, she'll go straight to Intensive Care. Let's go get a hot drink and then we'll find out where we need to go and wait for news there."

Simon, too, resisted at first, but with a little gentle persuasion from Alex and Beth agreed that it would be better to move, to do something, rather than just sit on those hard, plastic chairs with other people just as anxiously waiting for news of their loved ones or treatment for their own cuts and broken bones.

He allowed Alex to lead the way, and soon he, Anna and Beth were sitting opposite each other at a table by the window, clean but still damp from a recent wiping. Alex went to get drinks and snacks.

Simon gazed at Anna and Beth, marvelling afresh at how much his granddaughter resembled Sylvia when she'd been that age. Beth's huge hazel eyes were teary and bloodshot, her makeup was smeared, her hair coming loose from the band of her ponytail, but to Simon she was beautiful.

For the first time, he registered that it was dark outside. It was eight o'clock in the evening so five hours had passed since Sylvia had first informed him that she felt weird. It felt like five years.

They talked about what had happened, Simon telling them in as much detail as he could remember.

"I'm glad Alex was able to bring you here," he said to Anna. "I'd forgotten until you arrived that Felix is away. It's a good job Alex was home, I wouldn't have wanted you driving while you were upset and worried."

"If he hadn't been," said Beth. "I would've taken a taxi and picked Mum up. I wouldn't have let her drive, Pops, nor risk driving myself in the state I'm in."

Anna put out her hands and Simon took one, Beth the other, and they tried to reassure each other that all would be well, because Sylvia was a strong woman who'd hardly had a day's illness in her life. She would fight her way back to them.

Alex returned with a tray laden with four steaming mugs, sachets of sugar and a selection of plastic-wrapped sandwiches and packets of crisps and biscuits. They each took a drink, milky tea for Simon and Anna, strong coffee for Alex and Beth, and Alex opened all the packets and spread the contents out so they could help themselves. Simon's stomach rumbled but he didn't think he'd be able to take a bite, let alone swallow any food.

Alex wanted to know exactly what had happened, and Simon recounted again what he'd already told Anna and Beth just minutes before, but he knew Alex needed to hear it too. It was all such a shock, he felt even as he went over the events of the last hours that he was talking about someone else.

Sylvia had shown no outward signs of illness whatsoever in the days prior to this one, so how could she be having a heart attack? And her symptoms had not given him an inkling of how serious it was until she'd started clutching herself and rocking forward and back, forward and back. She had told him that her jaw and shoulders ached, and by the time the paramedics arrived she had clearly been in a great deal of pain and distress.

Then, in the ambulance on the way to the hospital, she'd admitted with a whisper that she'd been having palpitations for a few days and this morning she'd been woken up by what she thought had been indigestion. Simon had felt terror grip his own heart then, and he felt it now.

By the time the hot drinks had been drunk, or half-drunk in Simon's case, and he, Anna and Beth had shared a couple of cheese sandwiches, Simon was impatient to find out if there was any news.

As they walked back along the harshly-lit corridors, Simon felt something snap like a twig in his brain. He kept walking but couldn't think where he was, or why he was there.

A woman was walking beside him on his right, there was a younger woman and a tall, dark-haired man who seemed familiar were three paces ahead of him, but no names came to mind. The younger woman held hands with the man, whose shoes squeaked on the linoleum floor, and she turned to say something to Simon. She was looking straight at him, her mouth moving. He was struck by how much she looked like his Sylvia.

Or was it Sylvia he was looking at? His wife, soul mate, best friend.

Confused, he was about to ask who they were and what they were doing in this place when there was another snap and the confusion disappeared as full memory slammed back into his brain: the man was Alex; the woman on his arm was his granddaughter, Beth; the other woman was his daughter, Anna, and they were in the city hospital, because Sylvia was very ill.

Heart attack.

Emergency surgery.

He must be suffering from a panic attack. How else could

he have forgotten, even for a split second, what was happening to his wife in an operating theatre somewhere in this huge, imposing building?

***

It was a dream, yet not a dream. Sylvia, for the first time in her life, was lying on an operating table in a hospital. She could hear the monitors, the quiet requests of the surgeon asking for what he needed, the clinks and chinks of metal as a nurse sorted through the instruments and lined them up on a large tray, handing over forceps, scissors, clamps and keeping other surgical tools lined up ready. She wondered how she could hear it all and worried that the anaesthetic was wearing off. You heard about such things happening, where patients felt everything yet could do nothing to alert the surgeons that they were awake.

Terror gripped her as she braced herself for intense pain, but instead she came out of her body and was looking down on the scene.

She had a bird's eye view of the surgical team working on her, could see her physical self completely draped in green cloths. Only her head and chest area were exposed, her eyelids held closed by narrow strips of white tape, her rib cage cut through and spread open with something that looked like a medieval torture instrument. She could see her beating heart in the dark, gaping cavity. One gowned and masked figure asked for suction and another pushed a rubber tube into her open chest and there was a soft, gurgling noise.

She was a witness to all of this and yet felt nothing for the physical part of her that was laid out on that table, for somehow, she recognised it as the most unimportant part of who she was. It was merely a shell, the vessel that had held Sylvia Winston, Mrs Sylvia Savarese as she had been these past fifty-eight years. She was released from it now, yet it still felt like she was seeing with physical eyes, hearing with physical ears.

There was music playing; a light, soothing jazz. She searched for the source. Was it in the operating theatre or coming from somewhere else?

Her thoughts turned to Simon, who would for sure be able to identify both the music and the composer, and wondered where he was and how he was coping. He was due to have his brain scan; would he remember it? She had no idea how much time had passed, maybe he had already had the scan? Oh, she wished she'd told Anna what was going on instead of waiting for the tests to be done and a diagnosis given. Why did she have to so catastrophically collapse before she'd had the chance to sort things out?

Without knowing how, she found herself moving outside and away from the theatre, gliding effortlessly along a wide corridor with cold strip lighting and a shiny, dark blue, linoleum floor.

A thin, stooped man was walking away from her, pushing a clattering cleaning cart with a wide broom and drooping grey mop sticking up above his shoulder. She cried out when she saw that Alex and Beth were walking towards her, Anna and Simon following behind, but it seemed none of them heard her and they couldn't see her.

Anna and Beth looked almost childlike, she thought, they were both so much shorter than the two men. For a wild moment she wondered if Alex could see her, but surely not. She wasn't dead. Or was she? No, it was obvious that he did not see her, nor did anyone else walking up the corridor in the same direction acknowledge her presence. She floated right up beside Simon, managing to keep pace with him as she peered into his face. There was a glazed expression in his eyes, a tightness to his mouth, a look she had come to dread.

Oh God, what if she didn't pull through when he needed her so badly, when they all needed her? Would Anna be able to manage things? And what of her poor darling granddaughter, how would Beth cope with another tragedy after the grief she had so recently come through?

Why did Sylvia's heart have to cause all this trouble now, when there was so much she needed to do?

For the sake of her family she had to get back to her body. Get back to it and live.

Chapter 12

Alex and Beth didn't linger in conversation over breakfast as they usually did because they needed to get across town to pick up Simon. Two days earlier Simon had managed to damage his car by reversing into a bollard in the hospital car park and now refused to drive it even though it wasn't at all serious; he could still close and lock the boot and the car was perfectly okay to drive. It had really knocked his confidence though, so now they or Anna collected him and took him to the hospital, or he went by taxi.

Sylvia was showing no signs of recovery and Alex felt sad that Beth's world had painfully shifted yet again and she faced the heartrending possibility of losing her beloved gran.

Beth looked so tired, he hated seeing the dark shadows under her eyes again as she said she wished she could crawl back into bed and stay there for a week. Every time the phone rang he saw how she flinched and if it was her mum or granddad, she had to visibly brace herself to answer it and hear the latest news.

Yesterday, she had answered a call from Simon, who'd been at Sylvia's bedside all morning, saying that Sylvia was showing signs of waking up. Alex, Beth and Anna had rushed there in high excitement only to find Simon had misunderstood the doctor and their hopes had been raised for nothing.

Anna tried to get Simon to come away from Sylvia's room for a short while, to have a drink or something to eat, but he wouldn't leave her bedside, so Beth and Alex offered to go and find something for him so he could stay near her. Anna had followed them out, and as soon as they were out of Simon's earshot she said that she had never seen him look so haggard, and she was worried about his frequent memory lapses and refusal to drive.

"It was such a little accident, something any one of us could have done under all this stress, but maybe at his age he shouldn't be driving any more anyway? He's always been so sprightly I find it hard to think of him as old, but he's really aged since Mum's been in here. I want him to come and stay with me and Felix," she'd said. "But he point-blank refuses. I'm sure he's not eating properly, and he really shouldn't be alone. Beth, darling, see if you can talk some sense into him, will you? Pops won't listen to me at all!"

That was yesterday. Today was a new day and maybe, just maybe, Sylvia would come back to them after almost two weeks in a coma. Even the word stopped Alex in his tracks. How could 'coma' have anything to do with the lively, vibrant, young-at-heart Sylvia? Come to that, how could 'heart attack' have anything to do with her either? In the years he'd know her she'd not had a day's illness. Yet it was all too real and he had to help Beth and his in-laws deal with it.

Beth's mobile started trilling in her handbag five minutes after they'd started the journey.

"It's Pops," she told Alex. "I hope it really is good news this time."

Alex listened to the one-sided conversation.

"Hi Pops . . . what do you mean? Is everything okay? You sound annoyed . . . no, we're on our way now. Pops . . . Pops, listen to me! We're not late. No, listen . . . are you there?"

She looked at Alex in surprise and said, "He hung up on me! He says we're late."

"He just wants to be there as soon as possible; I'm surprised he isn't camping outside the ward. He's stressed, Beth, that's all. You'll have to have another word with him about going to stay with Anna and Felix, it would be much better for all of us if he did."

Clenching his jaw at the prospect of another distressing visit to Intensive Care, he wondered with despair why no-one at the hospital could answer why Sylvia had lapsed into a coma following the bypass surgery. It happened, they said. Neurological damage, lack of oxygen to the brain, adverse reaction to anaesthesia, and they used medical terms beyond the average person's understanding. They would keep conducting tests, they told them, and her vital signs were good, so no-one was to give up hope.

A light rain pattered the windscreen as Alex turned the car into the street where Beth's grandparents had lived for the best part of forty years. Her mobile started to ring again, and he could see Simon standing at the end of the driveway with his phone pressed to his ear. Was he calling her again? He tooted the horn as he pulled up to the kerb, and for a strange couple of seconds Simon looked straight at him with no welcoming smile on his face. In fact, he looked furious. As he pressed a button on his phone, Beth's stopped ringing.

They both got out of the car and Alex was relieved when Simon's face at last relaxed and he hugged her and warmly shook Alex's hand.

Beth spoke gently, "Were you ringing me again? I said we were on our way."

"I was worried. You're so late."

Beth checked her watch and told him they were, in fact, almost ten minutes earlier than they'd said. "So, are you going to get ready?"

"What do you mean? I am ready. I've been waiting for you!"

With a sidelong glance at Alex, she pointed down at Simon's feet. "You're still wearing your slippers, Pops."

Rather than laughing, as Alex expected him to, he heaved a heavy sigh of irritation and plodded back into the house. Within moments he reappeared with his shoes on and joined them in the car and Alex was happy to see that his humour had been restored as he said in a cheerful voice, "Maybe today's the day, eh? Paul's coming later. Sylvia's always loved listening to his voice. Maybe he'll be the one to bring her back to us, eh Beth?"

As he drove them to the city hospital, Alex mulled over Simon's quick-changing moods of the past few months and uncharacteristic tactlessness. After Simon's comment about Paul, Beth would be fighting against the exasperation and jealousy that stabbed her in the heart every time Simon held out the hope that it would be her brother who would make a difference.

The doctors and nurses said it was entirely possible that Sylvia could hear them so they all talked and read to her, for hours at a time, so it was insensitive of Simon to say that it would be Paul's voice that would be able to reach into the dark depths of wherever Sylvia had retreated to and not Beth's. Or Anna's. Did Sylvia really favour her grandson over all the other members of the family? Of course she didn't.

After long discussions and by agreement, the family had

held off calling Paul and Adele because they didn't want to interrupt their honeymoon, but when Sylvia hadn't woken up as expected the day after her operation, Anna had insisted that they be told.

"Paul would want to know," she'd said. "Adele will support their coming back early. If we don't tell them and Mum doesn't . . ." She'd been unable to finish the sentence, the thought of Sylvia dying simply incomprehensible.

"Let me call him," Alex had offered, and she'd been so grateful, saying that she wouldn't have been able to talk to Paul without breaking down. Far better the news should come from Alex, who would be able to deliver it calmly and succinctly.

Felix had come straight home too, and was spending as much time in the hospital as his job allowed. He told Alex how much he appreciated his support, and Alex had replied in turn that he could see just how much Felix's own quiet strength steadied Simon, Anna and Beth.

Paul had taken the news with characteristic stoicism and he and his bride had taken the first flight home. They were staying with Anna and Felix and spending what remained of their honeymoon haunting the hospital as much as Beth, Anna and Simon did.

Paul didn't show his emotions often, but he was as emotional once he'd seen Sylvia as he had been when Amber, his little niece, had died. Alex could also see that Beth, just like that harrowing time when Amber died, was not comforted by it. She preferred it when Paul was his usual self, rather arrogant but always endearing, covering his deeper feelings with sarcasm or silly jokes, not red-eyed, quiet and bewildered as he was now.

Sylvia had always been at the centre of their lives; none of the family could imagine life without her, and seeing the stress

Anna was under at the thought of losing her mum but trying so hard to be a rock for Simon only added to everyone else's stresses. As for Simon . . . well, he clearly wasn't coping at all, and that should surprise nobody.

***

Sylvia looked on as her family sat in vigil by her bedside. Simon held her left hand in both of his, turning her wedding ring and stroking her fingers one by one, over and over. Anna was next to him, reading aloud from the day's newspaper. Sylvia didn't want to hear what was happening in the world; she only wanted news of her family. How was Simon coping at home? Had he been for the tests and the scan? What did they all do when they weren't at the hospital? Why had Paul and Adele cut their honeymoon short?

She was at a loss to understand what had happened. One moment she was a spectator in the operating theatre as the surgeons worked to bypass the blocks in her struggling heart with veins taken from her arm and leg, the next she was watching Simon, Beth and Alex walking up a corridor.

She'd thought of returning to her body but immediately felt a tremendous jolt and found herself back in the theatre. Just reflecting on that had her back there now, like an action replay.

There was some commotion going on, but she regarded it all impassively from where she hovered just below the ceiling, impressed by the surgeon's skill with needle and suture but wondering how bad the scars would be. It took a moment before she realised that the body below—her precious body—had gone into cardiac arrest again.

The medical team fought hard to bring her back and she fought even harder to return to her body, but it proved impossible. She was shocked to the core to hear it declared that Sylvia Savarese had slipped into a coma. The lead surgeon had noted the date and time, peeled off his gloves, and walked out of the theatre.

A little while after that, she'd trailed after her own body as it was wheeled to Intensive Care and hooked up to various machines, machines that would keep her alive while they tried to work out what had happened and how to treat her. IV lines and tubes were inserted in various parts of her body, a ventilator forced air into her lungs, a cannula taped securely to the back of her hand awaited drugs to be administered, and sensors were stuck on her chest either side of the narrow dressing that covered the long line of neat black stitches, feeding their data to the monitor above her bed.

With a glance at that monitor she was back in the present, feeling even more frustrated. How could she force herself back in so that her body would function on its own again? What did she have to do?

It didn't matter how hard she tried she remained separate from her physical self and so had to endure seeing Simon, Anna, Beth and Paul weeping over her, reading to her, pleading with her to wake up.

She wanted to shake them, to yell into their ears that she could hear them, that she was in the room with them, but it seemed she was powerless to do anything other than observe, unheard and invisible.

Even when Alex was in the room, her handsome, enigmatic grandson-in-law who could talk to the dead, she could not make him aware of her presence. In fact, she admitted wryly to herself, maybe it was a good thing that he couldn't see or hear her, because it was surely proof that she wasn't yet dead!

She smelled Paul's strong, expensive aftershave moments before he arrived, worry etched into his tanned face. He kissed first Anna, then Beth, before hugging Simon. Anna asked if Adele was with him.

"We saw Alex outside as we came in," Paul replied. "He and Adele have gone to the café. It's a shame they won't let all of us in here together."

Sylvia agreed, it would be far better if they could all be here together, but the space around her bed was tight and the number of visitors rigidly restricted. Alex and Adele, not being direct members of the Savarese family, had little choice but to wait nearby, only popping in if one of the others left the room for any reason.

Felix flitted in and out too, never staying long so as to allow Sylvia's nearest kin to spend as much time with her as possible. She was grateful that he and Alex came so often, grateful that their warm, calm presence was so supportive to Anna and Beth. How lucky she was with her family, she thought.

Her partnership with Simon had been joyous from the beginning, their fall outs had been few and far between, nothing more than the usual minor spats between a happily married couple. When Anna had been born Sylvia hadn't minded that Simon had fallen so deeply and irrevocably in love with their little girl, because she felt the same. They had become a close-knit family of three until Anna had grown up and married Felix, and they had embraced him lovingly. A year after the wedding, Paul had been born and a year and half after that Beth had come along, both of them making Sylvia and Simon the proudest of grandparents.

Ah, the grandchildren. Felix, like Anna, was an only child and his parents lived abroad, so she and Simon had truly appreciated all the time they'd been able to spend with Paul and Beth as the only grandparents on the scene. Beth had brought Alex into the family, and now lovely Adele had joined them too as Paul's wife. She stopped her reminiscences there, wondering why she was thinking about it all now, and not wanting to relive the pain of losing their first and only great-grandchild, the agony of seeing how Beth had suffered. Paul was speaking and she brought her lapsed attention back to hear him.

He was standing behind Simon, keeping his eyes averted from the various tubes snaking in and out of her body. He was a little squeamish, she knew, but of course he must appreciate that all the medical equipment, intrusive as it was, was necessary to keep her alive until she could breathe on her own.

"Any change?" He asked the same question every time he came.

On the first day, when he'd rushed straight from the airport, he'd sounded hopeful, almost eager for news, but the passing time had brought no change and it had dulled his optimism. Today it was obvious he had no expectation that the news would be any different, and his shoulders sagged when Anna said they would be conducting more tests that afternoon.

Sylvia had heard the doctors discussing her, saying that some change had been detected in her condition and they were very concerned, and knew that Anna and her family would be very worried and frightened when they heard this.

Once more Sylvia tried with all her might to force her way back into her body so she could feel her husband's hand grasping her own, make her lungs breathe without aid of the machines so she could speak to them all, tell them she was okay. She wanted so badly to hug and kiss them all. But her efforts brought no result. In fact, she mused, she was feeling more and more divorced from that thing of flesh and bone lying on the bed. The very idea of it was heavy and restricting, and she'd begun to like the being of pure energy she had become since leaving her body.

"Sylvia."

The voice was in her head, but she felt someone behind her. She turned slowly, initially afraid of who, or what, she might see, but she relaxed as a soothing warmth enveloped and embraced her.

The walls, floor and ceiling of the room slowly disappeared as if being painted out by a brush held by an invisible hand. Sylvia reached out to touch the sparkling pinkish mist that was all around her, feeling as if she was floating in candy floss.

A figure was approaching, too far away to make out any features, but Sylvia could tell that she was unusually tall in stature and her voice, though very soft, was unlike any she had ever heard. The figure stopped and beckoned to her and one word rang clear and compelling:

"Come."

Come where? Why? What if she followed this figure, whoever or whatever it was, and couldn't find her way back? But wait... Did she want to find her way back? As the realisation dawned just how much she wanted to go to that tall figure she panicked, for how could she so willingly walk away from her family after all her struggles to re-join them? Oh my God! Was she...

"Am I dead?" Sylvia asked.

"Come."

This time the voice was right inside her mind and, as if tethered by an unseen but benevolent force, Sylvia wanted nothing more than to go where she was led.

***

"What if she doesn't wake up?"

Alex blew out a sigh. "It doesn't bear thinking about, does it? Simon would be utterly lost without her, and Beth . . . well, I don't know how Beth would cope, having to deal with another death of someone she loves so much. It's bringing back all the dreadful memories of losing Amber and she's not eating well and hardly sleeping at all. What about Paul? How's he holding up?"

Adele shrugged. She looked tanned and glowing with health, but her tension showed in the stiff way she held her head and her shoulders.

"He doesn't say much. He's using work as a crutch, of course, but, well . . . you and Beth both forewarned me and I've seen for myself that Paul does not readily show his emotions, but he does feel them, and strongly. And Alex, I don't know how to say this, but I'm so sorry you all have to face another tragedy. I never knew your baby daughter, of course, but since becoming an aunt to darling little Hope it breaks my heart to think of what you both must have gone through." She hesitated, and Alex sensed what she'd say next. "Do you still see her, your little girl? And Scott?"

He smiled. "I see my little girl a lot, because she's with my father. Scott, I don't see him, but I know he's fine where he is, and he's bound to be watching over Lily and Hope. I'm sure he'd come through to me if Lily was to ask it."

Adele put her elbow on the table and rested her chin on her hand.

"You know, my sister Lily doesn't say much, she's like Paul in that way, but I think she's come to terms with it, as far as one can come to terms with losing the love of your life. And her coping with it is thanks to you, Alex. I'm so glad you were

"Hello?"

Whoever it was moved in really close to him, but he couldn't yet tell if the person was male or female. He could feel their energy, but it was weak and soft, not at all like the powerful force he'd felt inside. He surmised that whoever it was, he or she was having difficulty communicating with him. If only his dad was around to strengthen the connection! He tried again to initiate a better link.

"I don't know who you are, but if you can hear me then please don't give up."

There was a sensation of a hand brushing the side of his face, fingers stroking his skin in an affectionate way, leading Alex to believe that it was someone he was close to.

He concentrated even harder, straining every fibre of his being to hear a voice, no matter how faint, how fragile. Still nothing. The hand remained on his cheek and Alex felt a different sensation now emanating from the person in spirit. A frisson of fear, soon replaced by puzzlement. Experience told him that whoever it was could only recently have passed over, and as Sylvia was still alive there was only person he knew who could be a likely candidate.

"Uncle Alistair, is that you? Is Dad with you?"

At that moment he felt the energy leave him, a hesitant and gentle withdrawal, but Alex had only seconds of respite before the energy that had struck him inside the hospital hit him again and he almost gasped at the sheer power of it. He forced himself to relax so his psychic senses could expand fully, because now he recognised this immense power.

"Hello Grace."

She inclined her head in acknowledgement and Alex wondered as he'd wondered a thousand times since his near-death encounter after the accident he'd been in with Scott Miller who or what this enigmatic figure was. An angel or a guardian of those in the Afterlife?

Since sending him back from the Other Side to make use of the psychic gifts he had been born with she had appeared now and then in his dreams, particularly at times of stress, but not, he realised with surprise, for at least a year.

She was in front of him now and he was not dreaming. Her eyes, black as the darkest night, were fixed on him and he found his own gaze locked onto hers. Her lips did not smile, her face was totally impassive. He wondered with alarm if she was going to take him back to the Other Side with her to help Sylvia pass over, the way she had done when his friend Scott had died.

Grace had allowed him to see and experience the sheer beauty of the spirit world before sending him back. At the time he hadn't wanted to return, for he and Beth were separated and he'd wanted to join his daughter and his father. But he was grateful to her now.

"Grace, are you here for Sylvia?"

Grace merely moved her head, her astonishing eyes never wavering, never blinking. Was that an affirmative answer? He asked the question again, but she was fading now. Fading and then gone.

Alex kept his eyes closed, breathing deeply and evenly, until he felt himself entirely back in the present, just a man, a visitor to a hospital, lying on a grassy bank behind some bus shelters, the sun warm on his face.

Chapter 13

After removing her homemade face pack with warm water, Kallie wrapped her newly washed and conditioned hair in a towel and quickly put on her long cardigan over her shirt and jeans to keep warm before hurrying up to her bedroom to dry her hair.

This room was so small there was barely room to move around her double bed and open the wardrobe doors, and although it would make sense for her to finish clearing out and move into her grandparent's room, which was much bigger, she couldn't bring herself to do it.

After Walter's death, Verity had said a couple of times that they should clear out his things, but they never even made an attempt as Verity had noticeably begun to fade day by day. Besides, Kallie rather thought that it had been comforting for her to have her husband's personal things around her.

Now, even after all this time, her grandparents' possessions were still there: the flower-sprigged comforter on the double bed, Verity's make-up, the silver compact and powder puff on the tiny dressing table, a bunch of bluebells, the flowers fresh when they had been placed there, now colourless and desiccated in a crystal rosebud vase on the window sill, Walter's old and well-worn slippers by his side of the bed, their dressing gowns hanging from a hook on the door.

The bed itself was strewn with clothes and shoes where Kallie went in every now and again intending to sort through them, but it always upset her so much she'd leave the room and close the door without making much progress.

She plugged in her hairdryer and sat cross-legged against the pillows, running her fingers through the golden-brown tresses and reflecting on her gran's love of having her hair done and how she'd taken real pleasure in dressing well and always looking feminine and smart. What a shame she was five inches taller and a size bigger than her gran, otherwise she could have worn some of her stylish clothes, most of them made so beautifully by Verity on her old sewing machine.

It occurred to her then with a bit of a jolt that she, a trained beautician, was letting herself go a bit. The face pack and deep hair conditioner had used to be a weekly treat for her and for Verity, but before this afternoon she hadn't done it in ages, had only done it now because her last client had cancelled and she'd decided to come home early.

Of course, her face was always carefully made up and her nail polish never chipped because it was important in her job, and she always wore a smart plum-coloured tunic with light grey piping and dark grey or black trousers when she was working, but she'd got into the habit of scraping her shoulder length hair into a band rather than keep it the loose, layered style that suited her face so well. It was too long now and she noticed as she dried it that she had some split ends, so she definitely needed to get it trimmed, and maybe a few highlights would be a good idea.

She'd also not been eating properly, relying far too much on microwave meals for one and tubs of ice cream, so it was fortunate for her that she had the kind of metabolism that kept her slim no matter what she ate.

"Gran would have something to say about you, Kallie Harper. Time to get yourself sorted out," she said to her reflection in the mirror.

Humming cheerfully at her decision to take herself in hand, she ironed two of her tunics so she would have one to wear for tomorrow's stint at Rainstones House and a spare in case of spillage or accident.

Thursdays were fast becoming her favourite day of the week. She felt she was part of an important team there, and the Day Patient Unit guests who came to see her—mostly for gentle massages with aromatherapy oils—were so cheerful and always telling her how much they loved coming to see her. Plus there was Kevin, who she liked enormously. He made her laugh, and it didn't hurt that he was single, good-looking and seemed to like her too.

Fancying a mug of milky coffee while she read the latest issue of the holistic therapies magazine she subscribed to, Kallie skipped downstairs to the kitchen. While the milk simmered on the hob she reflected on a couple of clients who'd come into the salon to have their nails done, a woman in her thirties and her youthful mother.

It was their first visit to Kallie and she had quickly seen how close they were from the way they finished each other's sentences and laughed easily together as they regaled everyone in the salon with tales of hilarious shopping trips and shared holidays.

On automatic pilot Kallie had smiled and made the

appropriate responses as she worked on their intricate manicures one after the other, wondering all the while how the two women would react if she were to tell them how she hardly even knew her mother and they barely spoke to one another. It had made her wonder just how long it had been since they'd had one of their stilted conversations on the phone.

About to pour the hot milk over a teaspoon of coffee granules in her favourite mug, a loud bang had her instantly on alert, ears straining. She thought it had come from upstairs, but couldn't be sure.

Pondering on the episodes of the TV switching channels, the phone calls with no-one at the end of the line, and the lights going off and on their own, her mouth went dry. She carefully put the saucepan back on the hob and walked into the living room. It sounded like something had fallen from quite a height, or a window had flown open and banged back against the wall, but there was no wind this evening. Creeping into the living room she grabbed the poker from the hearth and wondered where she should investigate first. Should she go upstairs, where she thought the bang had come from, or check out the back?

Biting her lip, she moved stealthily back through the kitchen to the bathroom, making sure that the windows were secure and the kitchen door bolted. Returning to the bottom of the staircase she peered upwards. The landing light was on, which gave her pause because she was pretty sure it hadn't been when she'd come downstairs. The staircase was always gloomy but she wasn't in the habit of having lights on where they weren't needed. Did electrical faults cause things to go bang? She really must call an electrician to come and check everything, she absolutely could not risk a fire in a thatched house.

Leaving the landing light on she climbed the steep stairs, more aware than ever how loudly they creaked. When she reached the top she glanced to the open door of her bedroom, then the closed door of the larger room. She decided her own room should be checked first, but it took no time to see that all was just as she had left it not ten minutes before.

On tiptoe, she moved across the landing to the other bedroom. After all, she reasoned, as she'd been moving stuff and beginning to sort everything into piles for items she planned to keep, those she'd send to charity and those she would discard, wasn't it possible that something had shifted, over-balanced somehow and toppled to the floor? She walked round the double bed but nothing had fallen. She looked out the window to check that her car was still there.

The skies were clear and bright, but it would be a full moon tonight, casting a silvery glow on the churchyard. It was a sight she found beautiful, not at all something to bother her like it spooked some of her friends. Why people thought graveyards, where people had been lovingly buried in consecrated ground, should be the source of so much fear at night was beyond her. If they were really under the illusion that dead people could rise from the grave and haunt them, then surely it was those buried in unconsecrated ground they should be afraid of.

She let her eyes rest on the garden wall at the spot where the graves of Verity and Walter were just over the other side, sending mental thought waves of love to her grandparents, telling them that she would bring fresh flowers on Sunday.

The bedroom was a mess, but as she quickly ran her eyes over the piles of clothes and shoes strewn across the bed she could see that everything was just as she'd left it the last time she'd been in here.

The smell of her gran's perfume was very strong, though, and she couldn't think why this would be. Crossing to the dressing table, Kallie let out a gasp of surprise, because the crystal bottle wasn't where it should be. Working so much with aromatherapy oils she didn't wear perfume, but the beautiful bottle and its contents was something she had no intention of getting rid of. Just the sight of it helped her recall lovely memories of watching her gran hold her finger over the top of the heavy crystal stopper and tip the bottle once, twice. Verity would then take the stopper and stroke it behind her ears and on her wrists, perfuming her pulse points.

When Kallie had been very young and allowed to play dress-up in her gran's clothes and shoes she had been forbidden to touch the bottle as it was heavy and she might have dropped it. But her gran had sometimes given her the stopper so she could dab herself with a tiny drop of the lovely floral scent.

The bottle was not there and Kallie stared in bewilderment at the clean circle in the fine layer of dust on the dressing table surface. The circle in which the crystal bottle should have been sitting.

She felt the first prickle of fear as she wondered if someone had broken into the cottage while she'd been at work; the perfume bottle was vintage, one of the few things Verity had as a reminder of her wealthy upbringing, and worth several hundred pounds now.

Rushing to the drawer where her grandmother's jewellery was kept she yanked it open and quickly scanned the rings, pearl earrings and fine gold necklaces and bracelets that were neatly laid out on dark blue velvet pads. Nothing was missing.

"Come on, Kallie," she reassured herself. "The TV is still downstairs, the laptop is on the floor next to the sofa, there are no broken windows and you had to turn the front door key twice to open it so there's been no forced entry. Nothing downstairs or up here has been ransacked."

No, she hadn't been burgled. She must have moved the bottle and just forgotten about it. Maybe it was in her own bedroom, or in the bathroom? It was the best explanation she could come up with, though it rankled that she could be so forgetful, and she was still no nearer to understanding what had made that tremendously loud bang.

As she walked towards the door the smell of *Joy* got even stronger, forcing her to look back nervously over her shoulder. A shadow moved by the dressing table. She would swear it.

Trembling a little, she turned her body all the way round and brought the poker up in front of her, gripping it with both hands as if it were a samurai sword. She stared intently at the dressing table and the area around it. Nothing moved, but as her eyes scanned the area she spotted the perfume bottle on its side beneath the dressing table. The stopper had rolled a couple of feet away from it, and perfume had spilled onto the carpet making a dark stain on the cream wool.

Blowing out the breath she hardly realised she'd been holding, Kallie relaxed her grip on the poker and slowly lowered it. The bottle falling to the floor would not have made the loud bang she'd heard, but it did explain the intense smell of *Joy* and why it wasn't on the dressing table: she had obviously knocked it over when sorting through the drawers and simply not noticed.

She retrieved the bottle, pleased to see there was still a little scent in it, replaced the stopper, and put it back on the dressing table, positioning it so it sat exactly in the circle in the fine dust.

Whatever that noise had been, she convinced herself it couldn't have been anything electrical and must have come from outside. It could have been something as innocent as a car door being slammed shut in the church car park or the lane, but because she'd been in such deep thought she'd not recognised the direction or cause of the sound.

The ringing phone summoned Kallie back downstairs. Would it be one of those calls where no-one spoke? She glanced at her watch, saw it was almost half past four. A friendly voice asked to speak with Miss Kathleen Harper and Kallie confirmed that it was she.

"And could you confirm for me please that you are a relation of Celia Harper?"

More curious than alarmed because the tone of the caller did not seem to indicate that she was about to deliver bad news, Kallie said, "Yes, she's my mother."

When she'd understood who the caller was and the reason for the call she had to sit down on the floor and ask for it to be repeated. The patient voice explained again that her mother had experienced a bad fall at her home and was in hospital with some broken bones and other injuries. She had been there for three days and now they were happy to discharge her. She could go home tomorrow morning, but she had to be released into someone's care. Her daughter's telephone number was the only one Celia Harper provided, so could Kallie please be there to collect her as she would not be allowed to leave unless accompanied.

In a daze and still trying to take in this unexpected and most unwelcome turn of events, she immediately called Rainstones House, relieved that someone was still in the office. She made her profuse apologies and was told not to worry, they would arrange for another therapist to take her place tomorrow.

She wondered if Kevin would be sorry that she wasn't there, then pushed the thought from her mind as she had far more serious things to consider now.

She reheated the milk and made the coffee, but then sat with the magazine open on her lap unread. How strange that only that morning she'd been thinking about her mother and pondering their difficult relationship, and now here was Celia, slamming back into Kallie's life in a most unexpected fashion.

Though she was reluctant to see her, of course Kallie would go to Cambridge tomorrow. What choice did she have? She knew it was about a three-hour drive away, but she'd never been there so she had better get the full address of the hospital and key in the postcode to the GPS on her phone. But when she got there, what then? What on earth was she going to do once her mother had been discharged? She hadn't been told what bones Celia had broken, but Kallie fervently hoped her injuries didn't mean she wouldn't be able to manage for herself.

She would take her mother home, make sure she had plenty of food, and be back in the cottage by late evening, and she would still have most of the weekend to clear the big bedroom and move into it. She sighed. Why was she worrying about which bed she was going to sleep in come the weekend? When she was going to have to drive all the way to Cambridge tomorrow, find the hospital, find her mother in the hospital, and then . . . what? She couldn't get her head around it so decided the best course of action was to put it out of her mind, go to bed at a reasonable hour, and make an early start to Cambridge in the morning.

It was gone eleven o'clock by the time she finally lay down and pulled the covers over herself because she'd become absorbed in a romantic film on TV, but despite the mysterious bang, the unwelcome phone call about her mother and the prospect of a long drive followed by having to deal with Celia, she fell quickly into a deep sleep until the alarm woke her at half-past six the next morning.

Chapter 14

Feeling a bit winded and smarting after a collision with a tea trolley being pushed out of a side ward, Kallie stopped at the first seating area she came to and rubbed her bruised shin bone. The woman had apologised, but Kallie felt ashamed of her own, rather graceless response, especially as it had been more her fault because she hadn't been paying attention to where she was walking.

Besides that, it was bad form to take out ill temper on other people who had nothing to do with the cause of your bad mood. She wished she could track down the trolley-pusher to apologise properly and explain to her that she was in a temper thanks to the nightmare journey to Cambridge in her slow little car, getting snarled up in heavy traffic, then having to drive round and round the huge university hospital car park to find a space, racing against several other drivers also searching.

She'd been grateful for the size of her car when a space became available, which the Range Rover ahead of her couldn't get into. She'd quickly and neatly reversed into the bay before another circling car could grab it, sitting for a moment once she'd switched off the engine to calm herself before going in to face her mother. Now that dreaded moment was just moments away, for Celia was lying in a ward just a few more yards along the corridor.

She forced herself to take the few dozen strides needed and entered the ward. At first, she didn't recognise any of the women in the six beds and hesitated; she'd spotted Celia's name written on the whiteboard by the entrance to the ward and all the beds were occupied, but she couldn't see her. Not sure what to do, she was relieved when a nurse came to her and led her over to the bed on the left-hand side, in front of the window.

Kallie wondered if the nurse had made a mistake, for she could hardly reconcile the image she held in her mind of her mother with the elderly lady that lay with her eyes closed and mouth open.

Her long, wiry, wild hair, usually held back from her face with clips, was spread out messily on the pillow, shades of dark and light grey against starched white cotton. Her left arm was in a plaster cast from elbow to knuckles, leaving swollen fingers and thumb free.

Celia had been provided with a pale blue hospital gown, one that fastened at the front with a bow tied at the waist rather that one of those horrid, undignified things that tied up at the back, and Kallie saw that her clothes, in the usual shades of drab green, beige and black, had been neatly folded and placed on a chair beside the bed.

Celia must have heard her approach, because she slowly turned her head and Kallie audibly gasped at the sight of the livid purple bruise that almost covered one side of her face. It was difficult to look at the blackened and puffy eyelid, stitched and crusted with dried blood, without wincing. Celia mumbled something, then her head rolled back on the pillow and she appeared to fall asleep again. The nurse came back then and beckoned Kallie to follow her to the nurse's station.

"There's no need to worry," she said. "Mrs Harper had difficulty sleeping last night and is catching up now that her pain relief has kicked in. I know it looks as if she's been in a fight but apparently, she slipped and fell down some steps, we're not sure where. Her wrist is broken but there should be no complications once it's healed, and her eye looks far worse than it is; luckily, she hasn't got any damage to the socket. She really banged her head as she fell, though, and was in a lot of pain and a bit disorientated, so we kept her in for observation just in case of concussion, and of course we couldn't send her home by herself anyway."

The nurse stopped talking, giving Kallie the opportunity to speak, but Kallie didn't know what to say, not even to correct the nurse in her assumption that Celia was or ever had been married.

"Right then," continued the nurse. "She's ready to go home as far as I'm concerned, but that needs to be confirmed by the doctor. She will need some assistance at home as she's going to have to be very careful of her wrist until it completely heals. Obviously." The nurse waited again but Kallie still said nothing. "Does she live alone, your mother?"

Kallie, not missing the slight emphasis on 'your mother' and feeling stung by the manner in which it had been said, nodded. "Yes, she does. And I live in Wiltshire."

"Hmm. You've had quite a journey to get here, then. Well, the doctor will be doing his rounds in about fifteen minutes and I'm expecting that he'll be happy to formally discharge her now that you're here, so if you'd like to think about arrangements for her care during her recovery and come back for her in, say an hour?"

Not knowing what else to do Kallie left the ward and went to find some strong coffee and a large slice of cake to fortify herself while she considered the options.

She certainly couldn't stay in Cambridge and she couldn't imagine having her mother with her in the cottage even if it was the best solution for both of them in the short term. She didn't know if Celia had any friends she could call on, nor if she could afford to pay for someone to look in on her several times a day and help her, for she would certainly need help. How could she prepare and cook food, wash and dress herself with her arm in plaster?

The nurse had said she'd fallen down a few steps, but with those injuries surely it was an entire flight of stairs she'd tumbled down? Kallie tried to imagine what it would be like to have a broken wrist, but she'd never been injured other than the odd cut to a finger or grazed knees so she really didn't know. She didn't, in fact, know very much at all at this stage.

She reached for her phone intending to text Rosa and ask her for advice, but stopped halfway through composing the message. Rosa was sick with the nasty cold bug that was going round and was probably in her bed feeling sorry for herself. Besides, this was her issue and no-one else's, so she must put her practical head on and deal with it.

Checking her watch to ensure more than an hour had passed, she forked up the last piece of coffee and walnut cake, grabbed her bag and headed back to the ward. It seemed even further going back than it had in the other direction, the building was simply enormous, and she felt as if she were walking the bustling corridors for miles before she was once again standing beside her mother's bed.

Celia was awake and sitting up, a couple of pillows piled

behind her back. She rolled her good eye towards Kallie as she approached the bed and said, "Take me home, Kathleen."

No hello, no lovely to see you, or, how are you? Not a single thank you for coming all this way, and she called her Kathleen, a name which Kallie hated and had discarded many years ago. She felt her temper rise and pressed it down hastily. Her mother was injured and in pain, she must remember that.

"Yes, I'll take you home, but what then? You know you can't stay there alone with your injuries, how will you manage? And I can't stay in Cambridge to look after you because I need to work." She sounded sharper than she'd intended, but this was the effect her mother always had on her.

"I will manage just fine. If you would be kind enough to . . ."

She was interrupted by the arrival of the same nurse who had earlier spoken to her, and disapproval was written all over her face. She must have heard what Kallie had said and the way she had said it, and her estimation of Kallie had fallen even lower.

"As your daughter says, Mrs Harper, you simply cannot be home on your own. You will be quite unable to dress or undress yourself with that broken wrist. You will need help washing yourself, preparing food, all the things we take for granted until we can't do them." She turned to Kallie. "Please assure me that your mother will not be left to fend for herself?"

Biting back what she really wanted to say in reply to this obvious criticism of her lack of daughterly compassion, even though it was the truth, Kallie found herself saying that she had already decided to have her mother come and stay with her in Wiltshire.

Her own words surprised her, because she certainly hadn't made such a decision until that very second, and her mother looked equally dubious, though she mercifully kept silent. If they were to start arguing, as they usually did, she wouldn't put it past this nurse to call in Social Services to sort out this clearly dysfunctional mother and daughter.

The nurse drew the curtains round Celia's bed with a sharp swish and Kallie, marvelling that the curtain hadn't been torn from its rings, waited in the ward while Celia was helped to dress in her own clothes. She could hear her mother fussing and objecting, the nurse's firm responses that she needed her to co-operate or she'd be going home in the gown.

When the curtains were swept back again, her mother was sitting on the edge of the bed, her arm in a sling, being ordered by the nurse not to move because she would need a wheelchair.

"A wheelchair? Don't be ridiculous. It's my arm that's broken not my leg! I'm perfectly capable of walking and I'll be just fine on my own at home too."

The nurse, the hospital gown bundled in her arms, flashed Kallie a quick smile as if she at last understood the difficulties she faced in caring for her.

"Mrs Harper, it is quite a distance to the main exit and it is hospital policy that patients be taken by wheelchair. Now, your daughter has your medication and discharge letter." She turned to Kallie. "I'm sure you won't want to travel all the way back here to have the stitches removed or for check-ups so I suggest you get in touch with own doctor's surgery and ask for advice from them. Ah, here's the wheelchair."

Celia was expertly manoeuvred into it and Kallie, still in a state of shock and disbelief at the whole situation she found herself in, followed the cheerful porter as he wheeled Celia to the main exit.

When she had paid the exorbitant fee at the ticket machine outside the exit doors Kallie realised with extreme irritation that she had no idea where she'd left the car in what was a very large car park. She scanned the area, trying to locate a memorable landmark, but she had been in such a state when she'd arrived ... oh, wait ... yes! She spotted a sign she remembered seeing, and leaving her mother seated on a sheltered bench, she set off to get her car, thankful when she eventually found it.

She drove round to the pick-up area and once they were both belted in, Kallie having to help Celia pull the seatbelt across and under the plastered arm, Kallie got her phone out and opened the GPS app. But then she realised, with an emotion that was a cross between exasperation, wry amusement and disbelief, that she had absolutely no idea of her mother's address. It had been Verity who'd sent the birthday and Christmas cards; Kallie hadn't even signed them.

Celia, recognising the dilemma, gave her the name of her street and Kallie quickly keyed it in and slotted her phone on its dashboard mount so she could see the map as she drove.

After what seemed an age driving along really busy roads with numerous traffic lights that seemed to go red as soon as she approached them, Kallie at last saw the little chequered flag on the screen and heard the female voice announce that she had arrived at her destination.

Celia instructed Kallie to park in a visitor's space in front of a modern apartment building with a plain brick facade, and it came as another surprise to Kallie to realise her mother lived in a flat and not a house. She'd never given it much thought, but she supposed she'd imagined Celia living in something similar to the cottage, or at least somewhere with a bit of character.

They went up to the third floor in the lift, Celia ignoring her reflection in the mirrored sides of the elevator. Once inside the apartment, Kallie admired how light and airy it was, despite the floors and every surface being piled high with books and papers. It was far from homely and Kallie could see that her mother never bothered with dusting and maybe didn't own a vacuum cleaner. She hoped the bathroom would be clean because she really needed to use it.

When she came back out, determined not to comment on her mother's lack of basic hygiene, she found Celia in her bedroom trying to take some underwear from a chest of drawers.

It was obvious that her stitched eye and sore arm were bothering her, so Kallie offered to do it if she would tell her what she wanted. Celia told her to get a suitcase down from the top of the wardrobe, which Kallie had to stand on a chair to reach, then she sat on the bed while Kallie gathered the clothes and shoes she wanted.

There weren't many things, and it cheered Kallie a little to see that, although they were drab, her mother favoured skirts with elasticated waists and loose, button-front blouses that would be easy to take on and off. She folded and packed the items neatly, then went to the bathroom to collect her mother's wash things in a small zippered bag that had been in the case.

All the while, Kallie expected her mother to raise objections to coming back with her to the cottage, but since leaving the hospital their desultory conversation had skirted round the subject.

Celia said she wanted to take some books with her, but she gasped and winced as she made an attempt to stand up and inadvertently jogged her arm. Kallie helped her, surprised at how light Celia had become since she'd last seen her. Her mother had always seemed so much larger than dainty little Verity and Kallie herself, but that could have been the sheer force of her personality.

Celia said, "Are you sure about this? I can't say I'm not

grateful because I have no-one else to call on to help me in my predicament, but we both know this isn't going to be easy."

She didn't sound grateful and there wasn't a hint of humour in her voice but Kallie was glad to have it out there at last, and agreed that it would not be easy, but that they would both have to make the best of it.

"Okay, it's a three-hour drive. It's time for your pain killers, which will be a help, and we'll stop on the way for something to eat, though it'll have to be quick because I need to get back and clear out the big bedroom for you because it's still full of Walter and Verity's stuff."

Celia raised an eyebrow as she said, "You haven't done that yet?" Then, catching Kallie's expression and seeming to realise how unsympathetic that sounded, she indicated her bandaged arm and said, "I'm sorry that I won't be able to help you much, but I think you'll feel better when it's done."

Kallie nodded. "Yes, you're right." She smiled at Celia, attempting to hide her trepidation at what the next six weeks would bring, and said, "And now I have a good reason not to put it off any longer."

Thinking of just how much there was to do, Kallie was concerned at the short time she had available to get her mother installed in that room, because by the time they got back to the cottage it would be evening, and Kallie had to go to the salon tomorrow. Telling herself she could only take it one step at a time, Kallie picked up the case, now heavy with books, and they went back to her car.

***

Kallie preceded her mother across the threshold and into

the living room of the cottage, clumsily manoeuvring the cumbersome suitcase and putting it down with a thump at the bottom of the stairs.

Celia followed behind, closed the front door and then stood in front of it as if awaiting further instructions. Sighing, for her mother had been like this since they'd left Cambridge, Kallie apologised for the chill and said she'd boost the heating a bit.

She eased Celia's coat from her shoulders, mindful not to jog her arm in the sling, and invited her to sit down. Her mother chose Gran's armchair, the one she'd died in, but Kallie wasn't sure if Celia knew that and she wasn't going to tell her.

Celia perched on the edge of the cushion with her knees and ankles together, her one good eye looking round the room, and Kallie was amazed again at just how different her mother's physical appearance was to Verity and to herself. For the first time she realised how much she resembled Walter.

"Well now!" exclaimed Kallie in a forced jolly voice that was the opposite of how she felt inside. "I need to go and clear Gran's room and make up the bed, so would you like a cup of tea? Shall I put the telly on for you?"

Celia said, "No, thank you" to the tea and, "Yes, please" to the telly, so Kallie switched it on and handed her the remote so she could choose something she'd like to watch. She had quite a collection of DVDs but had no idea what her mother's tastes in films might run to. She rather thought romance, which figured high in her own preferences, would rate very low on her mother's list.

She went to pick up the suitcase to take it upstairs, but, having more books than clothes in it, it was too much for her to lug up the stairs with its sharp turn at the top. Quickly, she opened it and removed the books, placing them in a tidy pile on the floor against the wall, her mother watching her with her one good eye. Able to manage the case now, she carried it quickly upwards, chewing her lip as she thought how hard the next six weeks or so were going to be.

They'd hardly exchanged a word on the journey back. This woman, this untidy, grey-haired person who looked more eighty-six than the sixty-six she actually was, was a stranger to her.

They had not been alone together since after Verity's funeral when they'd had that row, but before that? Kallie had to think hard. Really, had they ever been entirely alone together before that day? Very possibly they had not, because Verity had always been there during Celia's visits as Kallie was growing up. When Kallie had reached her teens and they'd had that heated argument about how she dressed and wore make-up and did her hair, then her mother's outright refusal to ever divulge her father's identity, she had declared she no longer wanted Celia to visit.

This had saddened Walter and Verity very much, but Kallie would not be moved. Celia had continued to come, for she and her parents still wanted to see each other, but she came less often and Kallie always kept out of the way. Verity had made a point of phoning Celia every other Sunday, half-past ten in the morning on the dot, but Kallie had not been interested in hearing any of the news Verity tried to pass on.

When Verity died, Kallie had really not minded that she would most likely be permanently estranged from her mother without Verity there to keep that tenuous link between them. But now this unfortunate circumstance had forced them together and only time would tell if they could form a friendly relationship with each other. And if they couldn't, well, they only had to put up with each other for six weeks. Just six weeks until Celia's broken bones healed, and then Kallie would take her back to Cambridge and they could go their separate ways again if that was how things had to be.

If ever there was a woman who should never have been a mother, Celia was it as far as Kallie was concerned. Rosa had asked her once if Celia had ever hit her or abused her in some way.

"Absolutely not!" Kallie had said but she had struggled to find the right word to describe their relationship. She'd tried 'indifferent' but that was wrong because indifference meant a total lack of emotion, and that had never been the case.

They'd got on well enough when she'd been a little girl, perhaps something like the way distant cousins got on, but mostly because Verity had always been there to smooth the waters.

Celia hadn't been at all happy when, at nine years old, her daughter had declared she wanted to be known as Kallie and not Kathleen from now on, and had chosen to ignore it. All too often, though, once Kallie had entered her teens, their encounters led to explosive arguments. The one they'd had after Verity had been laid to rest had been the last straw for both of them.

Ah well. It wouldn't do to dwell on the past. Better to put all that out of her mind and hope that Celia's stay would give them a fresh start and they'd find a way to be more like a mother and daughter should be.

Kallie put the suitcase down, opened the window for fresh air, and contemplated the piles of clothes on the bed.

Walter's things were destined for charity or the dustbin, so she stuffed his things into large bin liners and put the charity bags on the back seat of her car and the others in the wheelie bin. She then did the same with Verity's clothes and shoes, keeping back all the things she felt were too lovely to get rid of in a hurry. They would have to go back in the wardrobe and drawers they'd come out of until Kallie decided what to do with them. As long as there was enough space for her mother's few things then that would have to do.

Swiftly, Kallie carried the rest of the bags downstairs, placing them by the front door ready to take out to her car.

She hung her gran's good dresses, jackets, skirts and blouses on the padded hangers that Verity had always insisted on using, and put them away. As she paired her gran's shoes and neatly lined them up on the floor of the wardrobe, she couldn't help a wry smile at the chaotic way her mother treated her own clothes.

Next, she fetched a tray on which to load all the items from the dressing table and carried them through to her own room, then she cleaned, dusted, vacuumed and put fresh sheets on the bed, a clean cover on the duvet.

In just over an hour the room was ready and Kallie was hot and tired, but she had yet to unpack her mother's things and make them something to eat so she had no time to rest. Dinner would have to be something from the freezer and she mentally ran through what she had.

There really wasn't much in the suitcase, Celia being far more concerned with having a good supply of text books than outfits, so it took no time at all until Kallie had them put away, frowning at the dull colours and shapelessness of everything alongside Verity's smart, colourful outfits.

She draped her mother's plain nightdress and gown over the dressing table stool and placed her slippers beneath it.

All the while she was thinking incredulously that, just as she knew nothing about her mother, Celia knew nothing about her either. Or did she? What had Verity told her in those fortnightly telephone conversations?

She would find out soon enough, but she'd quickly have to learn what Celia liked to eat, what her taste in music was, though Kallie rather suspected her mother was tone deaf, what she read for pleasure or were those heavy text books that seemed full of scientific formulae and diagrams her pleasure? Did she like to take walks, go to the theatre?

On her trips downstairs she'd noticed that Celia was watching a documentary, a programme that described the forensic science used to solve crimes, so that was no surprise. She quite liked those programmes herself, so that was one thing they had in common! She hoped they'd find other things too.

She and her grandparents had rubbed along so easily together, and when Walter had died she and Gran, so stoic and determined not to be miserable, had soon settled into a contented routine with it being just the two of them.

When Verity had died peacefully in her armchair, which was just the perfect way to go in Kallie's mind, Kallie had dreaded being alone. But she had adapted, and although she missed her grandparents deeply every single day because she loved them so much, she was gratified to find that she was comfortable with her own company. So, how could she now share this small space with someone she wasn't sure she even liked? How was that going to work?

She heard a creak on the stairs and a moment later Celia was in the doorway.

She sniffed the air. "I can smell Mum's perfume."

Kallie started to tell her about the spilled bottle, but Celia seemed not to hear her because she carried on speaking. "I was born in this room. Mum hadn't wanted to have a hospital birth so she didn't tell anyone she was in labour until it was too late to take her there. The midwife wasn't happy as I was her first and she was so tiny they were worried she might need a caesarean. But I arrived quickly and with no complications. Did you know that?"

Kallie did know because Verity had told her. She had also confided how sad she and Walter had been that there could be no more children because both of them had medical issues affecting their fertility; she had been lucky to get pregnant at all, never mind carry to term. Kallie decided not to let her mother know that she and Gran had ever talked about such things and so mutely shook her head.

Celia came further into the room and looked around her.

"This house is so small and dark," she said. "And too quiet. That view of the graveyard never appealed to me, I was glad my own bedroom—your bedroom all these years, of course—didn't overlook it. That's why I've always lived in modern places, you get more space and light and I'm happier with a view of a busy street and the sound of traffic."

Kallie bit the inside of her cheek. If her mother didn't want to stay in this room she'd have to move all her stuff out of her own and that would take ages. She couldn't keep the edge out of her voice as she said, "Are you saying you'd prefer the other room? I thought you'd like to have this one."

Her mother regarded her steadily, and Kallie detected an angry spark in the one-eyed gaze, although it was difficult to tear her gaze from the swollen and garishly coloured lid of the other eye.

"Did I say that I'd prefer your room? I don't believe so.

As you have gone to the trouble of arranging this one for me, this is where I shall stay."

Feeling at a disadvantage having Celia glare down at her, Kallie jumped off the bed and went to close the window and draw the curtains. If her mother didn't like to look at the graveyard she could just keep them closed the whole time she was here, but her mother surprised her with a smile and her next words.

"I apologise. I did not mean to sound as if I was complaining. I have nothing to complain about, because you are doing all this for me and I'm sure you're not at all happy about it. But please believe me, I am very, very grateful and I will try to keep out of your way as much as possible."

Managing to give a small smile back, Kallie said, "I'll just take your wash things down to the bathroom." She grabbed the plastic zippered bag and sidled past onto the landing, adding, "I need to get dinner started, so come down when you're ready. I hope you like beef casserole and rice."

Before her mother could answer, Kallie fled downstairs and into the kitchen. She leaned on the kitchen sink, looking at her reflection in the darkened window.

They'd only been in one another's company for less than a day and were already rubbing each other up the wrong way. Okay, her mother had just made the most amazing apology, but how long would the truce last? She knew what her gran would say to her, for Verity's way had always been to go softly, softly.

She could almost hear Verity's voice echoing in her mind, saying to her, *"You're going to have to learn patience and tact, my girl, and learn fast. Remember my rule: always placate, never retaliate."*

Straightening herself and pushing her shoulders back she

went into the bathroom and placed the toothbrush and paste alongside her own into the holder on the shelf above the sink. The idea came into her mind that she'd enjoy a long, hot soak in the bath before bed to ease the tensions of the day, but that soothing image was quickly replaced with another one that horrified her: would she have to help her mother take a bath?

Chapter 15

Alex was only half-listening as the production team discussed a new back-drop to the stage for his television show. Various art boards had been pinned up and each one was being assessed as if it would be the end of the world if the wrong one was chosen.

He'd been quite happy with the one used before, just a plain, slightly shimmery silver wall that showed him up to good effect in the dark suits he favoured as he worked on the small stage. He could say so, he supposed, but who would listen? He'd learned pretty early on that they didn't like getting suggestions from outsiders, even if one of the outsiders happened to be the star of the show.

He tuned out while the discussion went on, hardly believing that something so trivial merited so much serious attention. He reflected instead on seeing Grace outside the hospital. Alex had not seen her again since then and still had no idea what her appearance could have meant. He thought it must have something to do with Sylvia, but she remained in a coma.

His father might be able to throw some light on it, but he had not made an appearance either and Alex could only assume he was still busy catching up with his brother. What were they doing over there, he wondered, and how long would it take before his dad was ready to work with him again?

He was brought back to the meeting by Virginia, a fairly new researcher on the Eselmont team, asking him a question.

"What do you think, Alex? Like it?"

For a moment he couldn't think what it was he was meant to like, then he saw the image of his stage with the backdrop coloured sky blue and his stylised signature in navy blue blown up large and placed diagonally across the centre. Wanting to laugh at the absurdity of it, he agreed that it was most impressive, avoiding catching Paul's eye because he would know Alex really didn't care about the small detail, and then the producer asked him how he felt about having some one-to-one sessions filmed for inclusion in the show.

"We're still figuring out the best way to do this, Alex. We could select members of the audience that you haven't been able to talk to and invite them to meet you on another date. Or we could invite applications for one-to-ones, though Paul says his office is already inundated with letters from people trying to get to see you. Whichever way they are chosen, we would conduct the sessions either in their own homes, or a neutral venue near the studio, whichever would work best for you."

After giving it some consideration Alex replied he liked the first idea, of selecting audience members who hadn't received a message during the initial recording, but he really didn't mind where the meetings subsequently took place.

"Could you do a couple immediately following the taping, do you think? Then we could set them up in your hotel."

Alex shook his head. "I'd prefer not to, though I appreciate it makes it easier all round. It's very tiring working in front of an audience for several hours, so I wouldn't be able to give it my best."

"In that case we'll concentrate on getting the shows taped, then set up sessions on future dates so you can do however many one-to-ones in a day that you're comfortable with. We'll edit them into the rest of the show."

Alex gave his agreement and then there was a pause, the only sound was the producer tapping his pen on the pile of notes before him on the table. Alex's psychic faculties came on alert as he sensed another new suggestion was forthcoming, one that the producer was wondering how to phrase.

Eventually he cleared his throat. "One of the team put forward this next suggestion, Alex, and Virginia has already looked into the possibilities it may offer. This article in the local paper gave him the idea." He handed over a photocopy of a newspaper cutting.

Alex scanned it quickly. It was a short article about the discovery of human bones wrapped in a sleeping bag six weeks ago during the demolition of some Victorian buildings in Manchester. When a digger had uncovered the skeletal remains all work had had to be stopped while police investigated.

Forensic testing and pathology had proved that the bones had been there no longer than ten years and the state of the skull indicated some blunt force trauma, so any further construction at the site was halted while an investigation into a possible murder took place. Thus far, the police had no idea of the identity of the person who had been buried, they had no missing persons reports that matched the height and build of the remains so couldn't check dental records, and no-one had come forward with any information.

The only clue they had was fragments of anorak, pale green

wool, pink denim and a pair of small, scuffed pink trainers, making it likely the victim had been a little girl.

Frowning, he looked up from the piece of paper in his hand at the producer. "And the idea is what exactly?"

Paul spoke up for the first time since the meeting had started, and Alex caught the excitement in his voice as he said, "The idea is for you to identify the body and find out what happened! Just think, Alex, if you could communicate with whoever this is . . ."

Paul was prevented from finishing his sentence by his ringing mobile, and Alex's started a second later. It was Beth. If they were in any other kind of meeting there'd be glowers round the table at the interruption, but everyone in the room constantly checked their phones anyway so no-one got annoyed.

As Alex and Paul excused themselves and hurried away, each to a spot where they could talk in private, someone suggested it was as good a time as any to take a break and they'd reconvene in fifteen minutes.

Alex said, "Hi. Everything okay?"

All he got in reply was a sob, and his heart sank. It had to be about Sylvia.

"Beth? What's happened?"

"C-can you come? Please, c-come to the hos . . . hospital. Gran's . . ." She couldn't finish the sentence.

"I'll be right there, okay? You hear me? I'm on my way! Paul too."

Paul was pushing his mobile into his jacket pocket and Alex noted the tell-tale reddening of his brother-in-law's eyes as he came up to him, saying, "Was that Beth calling you?"

"Yes, but she could hardly speak. What's happening, do you know?"

Paul nodded, his expression grim. "There were tests done this morning and now doctors are saying we should consider switching off life support."

Dammit. Why did they have to be in London when they were so urgently needed at the hospital? It would take two hours at least to get back there. With a quick word to the production team boss and a promise they'd be back at the earliest opportunity, Alex and Paul were soon hurrying out of Eselmont's offices to Paul's car.

"Want me to drive?"

Paul shook his head and went round to the driver's side. "I'm okay. Besides, I know London much better than you do. Did Beth tell you anything at all?"

"No. She was crying too hard. I'm so sorry, Paul, what a horrible situation."

Alex saw Paul's jaw muscles tighten and hoped he could stay focused in the busy traffic to get them to the hospital in one piece. He decided it would probably be best to stay silent, unless Paul wanted to talk, and was glad when Paul turned the radio on. Luckily, it was a smooth ride out of London and they were soon cruising on the M4 towards Wiltshire.

It was almost dark as Paul's sleek Mercedes pulled into the hospital car park, just as Alex's mobile rang again.

"We're here, Beth. We'll be with you very shortly."

Paul found a space close to the exit barrier and Alex had to lengthen his stride to keep up as Paul strode at high speed towards the main entrance of the building.

As they walked, Paul spoke over his shoulder and said, "She's still alive, isn't she? You'd tell me if she wasn't, right? I mean, you'd know."

His mind conjuring up that one appearance of Grace, an

event he had shared with no-one, not even Beth, he kept his voice low as he replied, "I really don't know, Paul. Let's go and find the others, then we'll know what the situation is."

As they entered the corridor leading to Intensive Care, Adele was heading their way, clearly on the lookout for them. When she saw them she broke into a run, straight into Paul's waiting arms.

"What's going on?" Paul demanded. "Is Gran okay? They haven't . . ."

"No, no, try and stay calm, Paul. I'm not sure what's happening, but a nurse asked to speak to immediate family members and took them to a private room. Beth came out briefly to tell me they'd been asked to prepare themselves because the doctors were considering asking to let them switch off Sylvia's life support and they want to know if she has an organ donation card. Anyway, that's when we called you. They've been left to talk things over and I told them I'd wait out here for you, and send you in, Paul, as soon as you got here. Felix is on his way, too."

Felix arrived then, slightly out of breath, and Adele explained things again for his benefit as they all walked together back to the ward.

She said, "Anna wants you and Paul to go straight in. Alex and I will wait outside."

Alex nodded. "Of course. We'll be right here if we're needed."

Paul asked where the family room was. Adele led him and Felix into the waiting area and showed them where to go. When they'd gone she visibly sagged and Alex put his arm around her shoulders and pulled her to him. All the time she'd been talking to Paul he'd been able to sense that she was holding something back.

Letting her go he said, "Right, so tell me now, what's been going on in there?"

"God, Alex. It was pandemonium. I'd just walked in and suddenly all kinds of alarms were going off and nurses and doctors came running, pushing us all out of the way. A nurse asked us to wait out here. It seemed ages before anyone came out to tell us what was going on, and then, as I said, they asked the immediate family members to go into that private room. They really only wanted to talk to Simon, as he's next of kin, and Anna, but Anna insisted that Beth stay with them and Felix and Paul join them as soon as they got here. I've not seen anyone since Beth called you so I've had no more news."

"How about Simon? Have you actually seen him today?"

"Oh yes, but only briefly because, as I say, I hadn't long arrived when all these alarms started going off. I understand that he came with Anna first thing, and Beth arrived shortly after I did. The poor man is beyond distraught and won't hear of the machines being switched off. None of them want life support withdrawn, but if the doctors think there's no hope..."

Alex sighed and gently guided Adele to a seat, taking the one beside her, thankful that they were padded and quite comfortable.

"It might not come to that yet, but there's no point in asking because they won't tell us anything as we're not immediate family. All we can do is wait."

Adele clasped his hand. "You're not keeping anything back are you? You'd know if Sylvia was dead, wouldn't you?"

"Paul asked me that. I don't think she is, Adele, because I don't sense her. But the thing is, she's being kept alive by machines. Maybe she'll breathe unaided if they do switch off.

We have no choice but to rely on the medical staff looking after her."

He leaned back into the chair and closed his eyes, silently reaching out for his father. Surely, today of all days, he would be there?

"I'm here, Alex."

His father's voice was heard directly inside Alex's head and he sighed with relief to have contact at last.

"I can't see you, Dad. Where have you been? I've missed you and was getting worried."

"I'm exploring with Alistair. We have so much to catch up on and there are things here that . . . oh, I can't even begin to explain them to you, Alex. But I'm here now, and I'm sorry I worried you. You don't really need me, you know.'

"I do, Dad! Apart from wanting to talk to you, I need you to bring Amber to me."

Now he could see them both, his dad and his daughter, a toddler now. She gave him a sweet smile.

"Dad, they're talking about switching off Sylvia's life support. Do you have any idea what's happening to her?"

There was a long silence and Alex presumed that Fin was checking on Sylvia.

"I'm sorry, Alex, her vital organs are shutting down. I can sense her, but it's very, very faint. Do you remember when you crossed over for that short time after your accident? It feels similar to that. She's here but not completely. Her time is close, though, I'm pretty sure of that. I know you'll be strong for Sylvia's family, and I promise not to stay away from you for so long again. But, Alex, if only you could see the wonders I have seen, the wonders Sylvia will see when she's here!"

Their communication was cut short by the arrival of a nurse

who told them they might be in for a bit of a wait and that the vending machine just round the corner had at last been repaired if they wanted a drink or snack.

* * *

Sylvia sat on the grass with her face tilted to the sun and her eyes closed. A light breeze ruffled her hair and somewhere close by a solitary bird sang its heart out, its notes so sweet, so poignant.

Since following the tall, enigmatic figure she'd been here, alone and content in this wonderful place. She didn't mind, in fact she enjoyed the profound peace and the freedom to move this strange dream gave her. So much nicer than the confinement of her hospital bed in the ward with its constant noise. She had thought intensive care wards would be quiet, but they weren't. Far from it.

She missed her family, but in a strangely detached way, for when she tried to think about them the details of their faces and their voices seemed to drift away from her. Time seemed not to matter here, and all the raw emotions she'd experienced after the heart attack to the moment she'd been brought here felt as if they had happened to someone else.

"Sylvia."

Her eyes snapped open and she gasped at the sight of the woman standing in front of her. It was the same one that had led her here, but now she could see her very clearly for the first time and her black, obsidian eyes drew Sylvia to her feet as she stared into their depths, finding herself unable to look away or speak. She waited.

"It is time."

Time? Time for what? With a start, Sylvia realised she must have been away from the hospital for ages. The last clear memory she had of being there was of Simon reading to her. There'd been an annoying sound, one of those frightening alarms going off, and some kerfuffle around her bed and she'd fallen into this dream. Was she still dreaming?

No. Now she was back in the hospital, the tall figure beside her, and this was a nightmare.

Sensing with horror that her kidneys, liver and heart were struggling to work, their signals to her brain getting weaker as they tried to shut down, she fought desperately to get back inside her body so her spirit could keep it alive.

But no matter how she struggled, just like before when she'd tried and tried, it was no good.

The lines on the monitors at the head of the bed began to jerk in peaks and troughs and then the traces flattened one by one. As minutes ticked on, she had no idea how many, she perceived that the only sensation she had through her strange connection with her physical self was the air being forced in and out of her lungs by the ventilator. But her lungs were tired too, they wanted to rest, to stop functioning like her other organs had, and the equipment she had relied on to keep her alive now felt callously intrusive.

She had thought that dying would be easier than this.

Sylvia turned to the being with the unblinking night sky eyes.

"Where are my family? Why are they not in here with me?" she asked the woman.

"They are not far. They will be back soon to say goodbye."

"Goodbye?" A cold trickle ran down her spine. *"I don't understand! You said I wasn't dead!"*

The beautiful face and fathomless black eyes continued to look impassively down at her.

"You are not, but it is just a matter of time, for your physical self is beyond saving. The technology can keep you alive indefinitely, but being tethered to a machine when there is no possibility of recovery is not living. If there was a chance, the merest chance that you could be saved, I would not be here. You cannot return to your body, but you have nothing to fear."

Sylvia was astonished how calmly she was able to take this momentous news. Why wasn't she hysterical? How could she stand here so calmly with her body in front of her, the chest rising and falling with the rhythm of the ventilator, when her family, when Simon, so badly needed her? She couldn't leave him, not now.

"Is there really no way back? My husband needs me! I didn't have time to sort things out. Please, I need just a little more time!"

"Your physical life is done. You will be shown how to have a new existence, and it is wonderful. I understand your concerns for your husband. But there is Alex. He is a good and special man and will help your family, as I will help you. Come now. It is time."

Chapter 16

Alex took his seat on the plane and buckled the seatbelt. When this trip was being organised by Eselmont he had declared that he would prefer to go by train, even though it would be a long journey starting at six o'clock in the morning with two changes along the way. Eselmont had offered him a first-class ticket but he had refused it, saying he was perfectly happy to take the first empty seat in second class and read a book and enjoy some time just being by himself.

He would get a taxi at the station to the location and meet up with the film crew who had travelled there the previous day to scope out the site and plan the shoot. But then Paul had scuppered his plans for a peaceful journey by deciding to visit his parents the day before, stay overnight, and travel to Manchester with him. There would be no crack of dawn starts or train journeys for Paul, first class or otherwise; he insisted that they fly out of Southampton.

"Why take four hours when you can get there in just over one hour?" he'd said.

Alex had wryly pointed out that Paul wasn't taking into account the drive to the airport, but Paul had shrugged and said he'd arrange a limo to take them, and Alex knew it would be no good arguing.

It was a short, uneventful flight, landing in Manchester slightly ahead of time thanks to a good tailwind. Alex handed down Paul's bag from the overhead locker before grabbing his own. Paul, as always, was in a hurry. He wanted to get through the domestic arrivals checks and find the driver that Eselmont had organised so they could get going straight to the film location. The same driver would pick them up and take them to their hotel afterwards, and be available for any other places they needed to be taken to.

Alex followed more slowly, looking with interest around the terminal concourse, at the milling crowds, the shops, the cafes and bars, careful to keep his psychic senses closed as he always did when moving through public spaces. If he didn't protect himself he'd be bombarded with information about those around him, begged by those in spirit to pass on messages to people who were total strangers to him. He couldn't cope with that, wouldn't dream of just walking up to and tapping someone on the shoulder as they went by and saying, "Hey, your long-dead Uncle Harold/John/Wilbert wants you to know that they're okay."

When he caught up with Paul in the Arrivals area, he had already located the driver and was standing with him by the barrier, waiting impatiently for Alex to get a move on. The driver took their bags and led them to the car, stopping briefly to pay for the parking ticket.

As soon as the doors had been unlocked, Paul was in, sinking into the back seat and immediately getting to work on his mobile phone. Alex simply looked out of the window, blinking as they emerged from the harsh strip lighting of the car park to softer daylight outside.

He was so deep in thought about what was to come that he didn't know how long they'd been travelling before the car turned into a street that looked like a blitz site from World War Two. They were checked by a security guard, who, with a curious look at the car's back seat occupants, directed them to where the Eselmont crew was waiting.

A well-built man with a red baseball cap visible under his hard hat, clutching a clipboard, detached himself from the others, coming forward with a beaming smile and a cheery, "Hi, great to see you again."

Alex grinned back and shook the proffered hand, trying not to wince as his bones were squeezed in a very strong grip.

"Hi Marcus. Good to see you too. How are you?"

"Oh, you know, busy, busy! But delighted you're back with Eselmont again, I just loved working on your previous programmes."

Marcus glanced at Paul who had his phone to his ear and merely raised a hand with one finger raised to indicate he'd be with them when he finished the call. Alex could tell he was talking to Marcia, and it seemed a celebrity that Paul had been after for some time had finally signed up for Paul's company to represent him.

Alex chatted to Marcus, a man he really liked for his perpetually sunny nature and his professionalism when filming. Marcus had been moved to tears when Alex had taken him to a private corner after completing a show one day and delivered a very important message to him from his late mother.

"The light is good this morning, Alex," Marcus said, leading him over to the rest of the crew. "We'd like to film as you take a look around, just to get some shots, but no commentary from you is needed. The digger driver who uncovered the remains is working on another part of the site now but we can fetch him over to talk to you, if you'd like. The detective leading the investigation wants nothing to do with us. He's a total sceptic, but we'll see if we can change his point of view, won't we? When he sees you in action, I think he'll change his mind!"

Alex made no comment. He'd come up against police officers before who didn't want to hear what he had to say. He understood their stance, of course he did. They wanted and needed hard proof, evidence they could see and touch, not information from a psychic medium like him. Still, his hit rate was excellent.

He'd proved himself in the couple of cold cases he'd been asked to work on, and so Eselmont had in their possession genuine police testimonials, and these had helped to get the authorities to agree they could come here and film as long as they didn't interfere in the investigation.

The investigating team had now finished with the area and had released it back to the developers, but the construction crews had started work on another part of the site. That meant that the burial area would remain uncovered for quite a while before they restarted the work there and filled it in, giving Alex and the Eselmont team plenty of time.

By now Paul was off the phone and Marcus led them to a small portacabin that served as the site hut.

"Hard hats, boots and Hi-Vis jackets are mandatory at all times, I'm afraid," Marcus said. "Meals have been arranged for all of us at the hotel, which isn't far from here, but if you want anything to eat at other times we can send a runner out. There's a fast food stand where the demolition crews are currently working; the coffee is decent enough but I wouldn't recommend the food."

Alex caught the look of distaste on Paul's face and couldn't help but laugh at the image of him tucking into a hamburger that he would declare either half-raw or ridiculously overcooked, covered in greasy fried onion, cheap ketchup and mustard in a plastic-tasting roll. His brother-in-law had very refined tastes.

Alex said, "We'll be fine working through, I think."

Once suitably attired to meet the health and safety requirements for being on a working building site, they left the cabin and walked across to a long and high pile of broken bricks and rubble.

Alex could see a block of houses still half-standing several yards away, with torn wallpaper visible on the exposed walls in some of them.

"This area was all Victorian terraces," Marcus explained. "It was marked for redevelopment years ago but planning delays meant nothing happened until now, and they started clearing the site for new housing about two months ago."

He walked them around behind the rubble to what had once been the long, narrow gardens at the back of the terrace, explaining that the end one was where the digger had uncovered the bones.

"Of course, all work had to stop and the police called in. The body had been wrapped in a sleeping bag, of a type used by the army, so I understand, and put in a shallow grave, making it obvious that it had been buried there not too long ago so was of no interest to archaeologists. Pathologists have the remains now and we're waiting to hear what they find out, though the police are likely to keep that to themselves while the investigation is ongoing. How much do you want to know, Alex?"

Alex, staring into the hole gouged into the dark earth by the digger yet not seeing it, brought his focus back to Marcus and told him he didn't want to know any more than what he'd just told him.

"I don't want to see any pictures, either, though I might want to see photographs of the recovery of the remains at a later stage when I've made contact with whoever this was. Tell me nothing more, Marcus, nothing at all."

"Okay. So, what now, Alex? How do you want to play this?"

Alex could tell that Marcus was excited and intrigued, but his senses also picked up that Marcus wanted justice for whoever had been buried here. It was hardly a big leap to conclude that this was a murder, otherwise Eselmont would not be going to all this trouble of getting permission to cover the case.

Alex asked to be left alone for a short while. "I know you need to film, but if the camera crew could please stay as far back as possible, that would really help. I just want to get a feel for the place to begin with, then I'll have a better idea of how I want to proceed."

***

As the greyness surrounding her began to dissipate, Flora slowly became aware that she was back once more at the place where her body had been buried. She'd first been pulled back here when the big digger had unearthed her bones, still wrapped in the big man's sleeping bag.

She'd hovered around almost constantly since, watching with interest all the different people coming to see, to dig, examine, measure, mark and photograph. She'd recognised policemen and women because of their uniforms, and then had come white vans and people covered head to foot in white protective clothing and masks that made them look like aliens.

Her bones, clothes and trainers had been removed from the dirt, labelled, put in plastic bags and taken away, she didn't know where. The people had all gone and for a while there had been nothing happening, then she had been alerted to activity near her grave again and had seen the people in jeans and heavy boots with cameras balanced on their shoulders.

She could see one of them, the one she'd heard called Marcus, who wore a red baseball cap underneath one of those hard hats. He had a camera on his shoulder, pointed at a man she hadn't seen before. He was dark-haired, with a nice face. A kind face. He was standing by himself on the lip of the hole made by the digger.

He'd been talking to Marcus before walking to the very edge of the hole, and something about him held her interest. He was tall and slender, his face smooth and handsome, not at all like the huge, scary man who had come crashing into the house when she'd been alone, waiting for her mother.

"I can see you."

For a moment Flora thought he was talking to someone else. Not one of the hundreds of people who'd come before had ever spoken to her. But he was looking straight at her. Could he really see her?

"My name is Alex. Will you talk to me?"

Oh, she wanted to talk to him, but she wasn't sure how.

"You only have to speak to me with your mind. Just think the words and I will hear them. I'm a medium, do you know what that is? No-one yet knows who you are or how you died, but you'll be able to tell me and I'll be able to tell everyone else. Will you start by telling me your name?"

Her thoughts were jumbled and still she didn't know how to

talk to this man. He seemed to understand, because he smiled at her and kept talking.

"No-one should be buried without a name. They're going to make a clay model of your face in the hope someone will be able to identify you, but in the meantime they are calling you Tabitha, because this street used to be called Tabitha Gardens. Did you know that?"

She thought about it. Tabitha sounded like a fancy name, but she preferred her own name. And going to the trouble of making a model of her face? How on earth did they do that? She was aware that she'd had very little schooling so was pitifully ignorant of so many things. But those bones, her bones, meant nothing to her.

She'd been quite happy in the other place and not at all happy when she'd found herself being dragged through the fog and brought back here when her body had been dug up. As she watched the whole excavation she'd felt like giggling at the care taken to remove her broken skeleton, care the like of which she hadn't really known when she was a flesh and blood person. And they wanted to know who she was?

She didn't know how she felt about all that, but she did know that she liked this man. Alex. A nice name. A friendly name she could trust. She formed it in her mind and sent it across the crater.

"That's right, I'm Alex."

She studied him, reaching out with senses brand new to her, feeling her way to him with her mind as he'd told her, feeling the connection as her senses met with his. She encountered nothing but warmth, kindness and compassion, something she'd not had much experience of, only from her mummy, and she liked it so she edged a little nearer. What was he doing here? A medium? What did that mean?

He definitely wasn't wearing a uniform, she could see blue jeans below the bright yellow jacket he wore, and he had no medical instruments. He wasn't digging with a trowel or taking soil samples, he wasn't scribbling notes or taking hundreds of photographs.

Looking past him she could see others with Marcus, one with a microphone on a long pole that looked like a fluffy grey animal, reminding her of the cat at one of the places she and Mummy had stayed in. Flora had loved that cat, because it curled up on her lap and let her stroke its lovely soft, thick fur while it purred. That, in turn, reminded her of finding the cat curled up on her slippers once, the slippers she'd loved because they were pink and girly and cosy, but they'd been left behind when she and her mother had been forced to make yet another night-time escape from trouble.

She turned her attention back to Alex and lifted her hand in a wave. He waved back, a wide and friendly grin that showed his even, white teeth. He really was very good looking. And he really could see her.

She felt something else besides compassion in him as their senses continued to unite. She felt sadness, regret. For her. She knew it was for her, and wanted to cry for the knowledge that someone cared. Someone cared about her, just as her mummy had before she had gone away and left her.

She felt determination in him, too, an iron will, and that he had come here for a reason that wasn't the same as all the others. The others just wanted to identify her and get the answers they needed so they could get on with their jobs.

What did he want?

She glanced down into the shallow pit then back at Alex.

"Please tell me your name. I can tell you don't like Tabitha,

but that's what I'll have to call you if you don't tell me what you're really called!"

She smiled shyly and whispered, *"Flora. My name is Flora."*

It sounded as if she hadn't said her own name for a very long time, but to Alex it brought a bittersweet memory flooding into his mind, giving him an instant connection to this little girl.

"Oh, I like that name! When I was a little boy, probably about the same age as you, my Granny Mairi used to sing The Skye Boat Song to help me to go to sleep. Do you know that song?"

Flora shook her head.

"There's a lady called Flora in that song." Alex took a breath and softly sang the lines, *"Rocked in the deep, Flora will keep, watch o'er your weary head."*

Across from him Flora was giggling.

Alex laughed too. *"I know, my voice is terrible, isn't it? Be glad I didn't sing the whole song to you! It's a story about a dangerous sea journey, and this lovely lady Flora is keeping someone very special safe from harm. Will you talk to me, Flora? It would help to tell your story, it really would. And then you can go back to the lovely place you've come from and never need to come back here again. It is lovely over there, isn't it?"*

She wondered how he knew that, about the warm place where there were angels and everything was pretty. She thought for a long moment. To tell him would mean remembering the whole thing, but didn't she do that often anyway?

When she had died she'd gone straight to this wonderful place, a garden of light and warmth, but every time she remembered being shoved backwards and falling and hurting her head it was as if her thoughts caused the thick, grey fog to form. It wrapped around her like a blanket until she shrugged off the memories, and then it disappeared and she was back on the green lawn surrounded by flowers again.

Sometimes, she heard voices calling out to her, soft voices that carried love and caring, and she wanted to go to them, but the grey fog would close in again and she didn't know where to go.

All right, she would tell him.

She described her life, her not very happy life. Being dragged from place to place, living with men for as long they tolerated having a 'brat' hanging around, her mummy stealing food and clothes, something Flora hated her doing but Mummy had said there was no other way as she had so little money.

She described how they had broken into the abandoned house that had once stood here and the night they had spent on a horrible, musty-smelling mattress. Of her mummy going out in the pouring rain to get some food and Flora falling back to sleep, then waking up again, shivering, teeth chattering, scared because her mummy hadn't come back.

She'd been told not to leave the room, but she'd heard sounds downstairs and thought it was her mummy. She described the strange taste of the piece of cold and congealed pizza, the delicious taste of the fresh, cold milk.

"And then the man came. He was very big. He had a scarred face. I thought he was angry to find me there, touching his things. But I hadn't stolen anything. Only the pizza and a little milk. I was trying to run, to get out of the house and find Mummy. I'd thought that she had brought all the things in there, that she would light the fire and we would sit in front of it. I ran straight into him, that man, knocking the wind out of him and he pushed me away. I fell against the fireplace, hitting my head on the corner. The man was so very sorry, he hadn't meant to push me so hard,

but I had frightened him. I could hear him talking to me, trying to get me up off the floor, but I felt funny and couldn't talk. He hadn't been angry with me, he'd been scared! He told me that over and over and then everything went black."

Alex shook his head in sorrow at her tale, and Flora felt strangely relieved to have shared it with him.

"So, it was an accident, the way you died? The big man didn't mean to hurt you?" Alex asked.

"No, he really didn't. He cried so much and he didn't know what to do. He was going to leave me there, I think, but then he didn't want to because of the mice and rats, so he wrapped me in his sleeping bag and put me in the ground. When he carried me outside in the rain I saw him start to dig the hole, and then I wasn't there anymore. I wasn't scared. I was in a different garden and the sun was shining."

Chapter 17

This was the most peaceful place Sylvia had ever known, a place where she could quite believe the most damaged and broken of souls could be repaired. Her own soul was intact and she was grateful for that, she was merely surprised and confused about her new state of being and sad at leaving her family.

The tall being with the impassive face and astonishing black eyes had commanded her to follow, and she'd tried to tell those sitting at her bedside that she had to leave them, but no-one had heard her. Even Alex, who she was sure had sensed her presence and felt her touch on his face that time as he lay on the sunny grass bank outside the hospital, had not understood that it was her trying to communicate with him. He had thought it was someone else—an uncle? Sylvia couldn't remember.

There was no sign now of the angel—she could not think of her as human and angel seemed the most appropriate word—who had summoned her away from the panic and noise of the alarms, away from her deathbed, so she waited on the cool, lush grass of a vast lawn that spread around her as far as the eye could see, thinking about her family.

How were Simon, Anna, Beth and Paul coping? Were they looking after each other? Was Felix taking care of Anna and Alex looking after Beth, both of whom would feel Sylvia's loss so deeply?

Thank goodness Paul had Adele by his side now. Her deepest concern was for Simon. She had no idea if any other others were aware that he had a problem, that he might have a brain tumour or dementia. Had he been for the brain scan?

She had many questions about them, but also about herself, only those were so immense she couldn't dwell on them for long. She was dead and she hadn't expected it to be like this. It was just like a dream, and in the way of dreams the lawn had shrunk while she'd let her mind wander and she was now sitting beneath an oak tree, resting comfortably against its warm, solid trunk.

She slowly became aware of feeling an energy pulsing against her back and instinctively knew it to be the tree's life force. Her own energy began to synchronise with the pulse and she sighed with contentment.

Before her was a beautiful landscaped garden surrounded by beds of lush shrubs and vibrant flowers. Their perfume and sweet birdsong filled the air. Tinkling water could also be heard close by, although she couldn't see a stream or a fountain from her vantage point. The warmth of the day was pleasant and soothing, but the disc hanging low in the sky was not like the sun. There was a purplish haze over and around it, so she could look straight at it and not have her eyes dazzled.

Yes, it was like a dream state and it was so lovely, so restful, she wanted to stay here for a little while. But the scene changed again and she became aware that there were many other people in the garden, standing around in groups or alone. They hadn't been there just moments before so who were they and where had they come from? Why had they invaded her garden to disturb her peace?

She rose to her feet and headed towards the nearest group, but she didn't recognise anyone and no-one acknowledged her. They talked in low voices, but not in languages she understood so she walked on, stopping within hearing distance of each group, or moving close to individuals standing apart.

No-one seemed to notice her at all until one young woman, skin the colour of milky coffee and a thick plait of blue-back hair hanging down her back, looked at her with enormous, thickly-lashed brown eyes and spoke a stream of lilting words. They meant nothing to Sylvia, but the woman's expression and the intonation of her voice indicated that the woman had asked a question.

Sylvia shook her head. *"I don't understand you. I'm sorry."*

The woman frowned, gesticulating with her hands as she talked rapidly, not taking her eyes from Sylvia's face.

Sylvia shook her head again and smiled. *"I don't know who you are or where you're from. Maybe you're like me, new to all this?"*

The woman turned from her and hurried away, trying to catch up with one of the groups. Her feet were bare, Sylvia noticed, with brown swirly patterns painted on them.

She heard the metallic chinking of bracelets and bangles, and then noticed that everyone else was moving purposefully in the same direction. Incredibly tall figures with dark eyes appeared amongst them as if from nowhere, laying slender, long-fingered white hands on shoulders, murmuring softly to the people they seemed to be guiding. They were just like the one she had seen in the hospital. The angel who had come for her.

Sylvia found herself caught up amongst the milling crowd and so had no choice but to go with them. But she was curious now as to where they would take her, so she willingly fell into step and marched forward with the throng of strangers.

And then they were gone.

Incredulous, Sylvia swung around in a full circle, but she was totally alone. A little frightened she decided to go back the way she had come, to the safety of the great oak tree, but when she turned about she was further astonished to find that her way was barred by a high stone wall. Running to it, then going first to the left and then doubling back to the right she eventually came to a wrought iron gate set in a high Gothic archway.

A large padlock secured the ends of a heavy chain which was looped through the bars of the gate and a metal ring set into the wall. She peered through the bars, half expecting the view in that direction to have changed as well, but the garden stretched away in the distance, the great oak tree she'd sat beneath just visible on the horizon. She once more contemplated the high wall and the gate. Why had she conjured up a barrier? Barriers were meaningful in dreams, she was sure, but this was not a dream.

From somewhere behind her came sounds of young children at play drifting on the cool breeze and for the first-time thoughts of her great-granddaughter came flooding into her mind.

Oh Amber, she thought, *your time was so short would you even know me? Are you somewhere in this place or have you moved on elsewhere?* As the words formed inside her head she felt a tug in the region of her solar plexus, a tug that wanted her to go and find the source of that lovely sound of happy children. But she was distressed by the gate, not liking that her way back was firmly held closed by that chain and padlock. It didn't look or seem right to have such an obstruction here, and she pulled at it with frustration.

She peered through the gate again, longing to be back under the tree, but her view was suddenly blocked by the appearance of a man who seemed to materialise from nowhere. He stood with his back to her, but she knew who it was.

"Simon!" she yelled, shaking and rattling the gate. *"Simon! Over here!"*

The man turned, and she had to hold back a sob at the look of utter confusion on his face.

What was he doing over there? She called over and over again, shouting until she was hoarse, but Simon didn't see her and in the space of a mere second he had vanished. One moment there, the next not there.

Bewildered, Sylvia spun about begging for help, then she swung back to the gate.

"I need to be over there!" she shouted. *"I need to be with my husband!"*

To her amazement the chain fell apart and the padlock dropped to the ground. She pushed the gate open and gingerly took a step forward, her eyes fixed on the place Simon had been standing just moments before. Another step. She felt she was doing a momentous thing, but had not the slightest idea what it might lead to. All she knew was she needed to be on this side of the wall.

Hoping she would catch up with Simon she started to run, but slowly the realisation crept over her that she would not find him. What she needed to do was wait for him, for she knew deep in her soul that he would return. She went back to the tree and curled up beneath its spreading branches, her hand caressing its rough bark.

She was no longer a purely physical creature, she was—what? She felt like she still had her body, that she was still Sylvia Savarese who had all five physical senses, but she also felt so much more.

She lay beneath the oak for a long while but no-one came and eventually peace settled over her once again. She let herself relax, listening to the birdsong and the rustling of warm, scented breezes in the leaves of the great tree, until she fell asleep.

Chapter 18

Sylvia awoke from a dreamless sleep, feeling refreshed. She stretched herself and the daisies on the lawn immediately drew her onto the lush grass. Humming, she picked several handfuls and started making a chain as she had when she'd been a young girl. She had woven about half a dozen when she saw a young girl approaching her, her step slow and unsure.

The girl stopped several feet away, her eyes on Sylvia's hands as she pierced holes with her thumbnail and threaded the flowers together.

Sylvia smiled, and started singing, *"Daisy, Daisy, give me your answer do."* She glanced up every now and then as the shy little girl inched nearer.

"Want to join in?" asked Sylvia, waving her hand over the small pile of daisies beside her. *"My name is Sylvia. Why don't you come and sit with me?"*

The girl hesitated, her eyes flicking between Sylvia and the threaded flowers on her lap, then she came all the way forward and sat down cross-legged.

Sylvia picked up the daisy chain she'd made and added a

few more before joining the ends to make a garland. Placing it over the little girl's head she asked, *"What's your name?"*

"Flora."

"Well now, Flora, with a pretty name like that you must just love flowers! In Roman times Flora was the goddess of flowers and spring. Have you ever made a daisy chain?"

Flora, still a little hesitant, shook her head, causing her silky hair to swing forward, almost covering her face.

Sylvia selected two daisies and held them up. *"Okay, watch me do a few and then maybe you'd like to make me a garland to match the one I just gave to you, because a daisy chain is a sign of friendship."*

Ensuring Flora had a clear view, Sylvia began to show her what to do.

"See? You pierce the stalk about halfway down, like so. Then you take the next daisy and push the end into the slit all the way through so the flower head rests on the slit. Got it? You go ahead and do some then, and when we've used up this little pile we can go and pick some more."

They worked companionably in silence, Sylvia sensing that Flora did not yet want to talk to her. But she wondered where the little girl had come from and why she had wandered into Sylvia's garden. It didn't take long before the heap of flowers she had picked were almost used up, so she pointed to a large patch of daisies and suggested Flora replenish their pile. She went skipping off, her shiny hair swinging.

Sylvia felt someone approaching from behind her and intuition told her who it was. Shielding her eyes she could only see a dark silhouette, but the height, the graceful stride and the flowing robes were enough to know that it was, indeed, the angel.

When she came level with Sylvia she stopped, but Flora

seemed not to be aware of her for she carried on daintily picking daisies, making sure to pick the whole stem of each flower as Sylvia had told her. Sylvia followed the black gaze, startled to see that the child had suddenly moved quite a distance away.

Grace seemed to read Sylvia's concern and reassured her. Her voice, spoken rather than implanted into Sylvia's mind, was like music. *"Do not worry. She can come to no harm here."*

"But why is she so much further away? And why does she look like that... So slow in her movements?" Sylvia fancied she could hear the little girl humming a nursery rhyme, like a record being played at a very slow speed.

"I wish for her to take longer at her task so I may speak with you."

Sylvia stared up at the enigmatic being, the angel, whose great height from Sylvia's seated position made the difference between them seem immense.

"Who are you?" she asked.

The woman elegantly folded her limbs until she, too, was sitting on the ground, her robes spread around her.

"I am Grace."

Sylvia waited, hoping to hear more, but Grace was still watching Flora, giving Sylvia an opportunity to study her at close quarters. Yes, this was the one who had been with Sylvia in the hospital, the one who had brought her here. She had human features, but for her eyes. Her eyes were the strangest Sylvia had ever seen, black as black can be, with sparkles in their depths that gleamed like stars.

"Flora is waiting," said Grace at last. *"Just as you are waiting, because you both feel you have something to do before you can fully cross over. I brought her to you because she need not be alone and as you have a connection I wonder if you would be so good as to care for her until you are both ready to move on."*

Sylvia couldn't figure out what the connection between her and Flora could possibly be. There was no family resemblance, and Sylvia coming from such a close-knit family was sure she'd know of this child. How had she died? Why would she not cross over?

Her reflections suddenly ground to a halt in her mind as she registered what Grace had just said about waiting. She'd had that thought, that awareness that she needed to wait, and it sounded as if she was correct. Is that why she had felt so strongly about which side of the wall she was on?

The fathomless eyes fixed on her.

"Tell me why you are here, Sylvia." With a sweep of her pale hand she indicated the gate set in the high wall behind them. *"You were on the other side of it not so long ago, but the power of your determination to return here released the gate and you came back to this side. Tell me why."*

"I saw my husband."

Sylvia waited, hoping Grace might make some acknowledgement or give some explanation, but neither was forthcoming.

"I saw Simon and I just knew I had to be here, to wait here, for when he comes again. And I know he will come again. Why was he here so fleetingly? Did I dream it?"

Grace still gave no reaction, but Sylvia's mind was whirling now and for the first time she allowed herself to really think it through. She had unfinished business with Simon but what could she do for him from here? How could she make sure he was getting the help he needed? And how come she'd seen him here and knew he would come back?

As if she'd heard and comprehended Sylvia's thoughts, Grace asked, *"Do you understand yet?"*

Sylvia sighed and shook her head.

"I rather suspect that you know," she said, slowly. *"Are you going to tell me?"*

"I do not explain, I only guide."

Grace looked away from Sylvia and directed her unblinking night eyes towards Flora, still happily picking daisies in ultra-slow motion, before returning her alien gaze to Sylvia. Sylvia felt hot under the scrutiny.

Grace said, *"I told you that I had brought Flora to you because you have a connection. That connection is the husband of your granddaughter."*

"Alex?"

"When I first came for you, in the hospital, you briefly saw and touched him before leaving with me. Do you remember?"

Sylvia said that she remembered it clearly, how she'd seen Alex stretched out on the dry grass behind the bus shelters. She had no idea how, but she had been able to touch his handsome face, and he had responded but he not known it was Sylvia.

She had not thought of him since, her mind being full solely of Simon, Anna, Beth and Paul. But why on earth hadn't she tried to make contact with Alex again, to tell him that she was worried about Simon? He could have passed on the information to Anna, and Anna would have ensured Simon had the tests and got the medical help he needed.

She wanted to slap herself with exasperation; she must have been lulled into stupor by this place not to think beyond that first and only sight of Simon. That's why she was here, she needed to communicate to her family that something was wrong with Simon so they could get him treated! She had her answer, but now she also had a thousand questions. However, Grace had made it clear she would give no answers. What had she said? She did not explain, only guide? Something like that, so asking would get her nowhere clearly.

"I will tell you this," said Grace. *"For telling you will have no effect on the outcome for Flora. Alex is communicating with her, helping her to resolve what happened to her. He is the connection between you both and why I brought her here to ask you to watch over her for a while. She has been at her own waiting place, entirely alone, for a long time. She holds information about her death that she needs someone to know, and that someone also needs to give an explanation to her. Alex is going to help her, as he can help you."*

"Oh my God, how did she die?"

Horrified at the idea that something dreadful had happened to the little girl she paused, hoping Grace would at least tell her something.

"Fine, you do not explain, and maybe I am jumping to the worst of conclusions, but I don't know how to reach out to Alex! When I touched him he didn't know it was me, he thought it was someone else."

Grace smiled, the first time her impassive face had moved other than speaking, and Sylvia almost cried at the sheer beauty of it.

"As I said, that little girl over there speaks to him. She trusts him and they communicate almost every day," Grace said, rising with a graceful, fluid movement to her great height.

Sylvia started to ask another question, but Grace was already walking away and Flora had skipped back, her hands full of daisies. She so wanted to run after Grace and demand answers to the many questions she had, but Flora needed her now. She opened her arms and embraced the little girl, loving how the heart-shaped face grinned up at her with love and trust. It reminded her so much of playing like this with

Anna when she'd been little, and then with Beth, so proud to have a beautiful daughter and granddaughter. Fighting back the tears so as not to frighten Flora, Sylvia wondered how her family were coping and wondered, too, when Simon would come back again.

Chapter 19

Alex, Marcus and Virginia craned their necks to look all the way up at the East London high rise as they headed for the entrance, hoping there would be a working lift. There wasn't. Virginia offered to carry what she could and the men set to lugging between them the heavy box of recording equipment.

Slowly, they worked their way upwards, stopping for a breather halfway, Marcus moaning that the place smelled like a public toilet that hadn't been cleaned in years.

When they at last reached the twelfth floor they had to negotiate a long balcony open to the elements and strewn with abandoned bikes, skateboards and a couple of used cat litter boxes, until they were standing outside a scratched and battered half-glazed door. They were all out of breath.

Marcus said, "Remind me again, Virginia, why this couldn't be done in a hotel?" He removed his red baseball cap and wiped his forehead.

Virginia, puffing out her reddened cheeks, grinned. "Now I thought you were a super-fit gym bunny, so why are you complaining? That was nothing more than a light workout for you!" Her grin faded as she explained, "Rachel suffers from panic attacks and only goes out if she absolutely has to, usually for food and she goes in the dark. She insisted we do the interview here, where she feels most comfortable, and I had no choice but to agree."

She rang the doorbell.

Alex listened to it reverberate inside the flat, an electronic rendering of a tune he couldn't identify. A figure appeared, blurred by the frosted glass panel, until the door was pulled open to reveal a skinny woman with fair, shoulder length hair hanging loose and straggly. She had a centre parting which showed a good two inches of grey. Her eyes were shadowed. Haunted.

Virginia, who'd met her before when she set up the interview, introduced Alex and Marcus and asked rather anxiously if she was still willing to be filmed. The look she gave the three of them spoke a thousand words and Alex half expected her to close the door in their faces and send them back down those twelve flights of stairs empty-handed, but she stood back, and Virginia led the way in.

The flat hardly smelled much better than the stairwell, and the four of them had to cram into the tiny sitting room. Sparsely furnished, there was only a small cabinet in the corner, one armchair and a sagging couch with an arm missing. The mismatched fabric of both was faded, stained and ripped in places where the material had worn thin. The only other seat was a dark green plastic garden chair. The walls were unbroken by pictures or hangings of any kind, the thin curtains were too short, the carpet threadbare, and everything was in varying shades of grey. Even the damp stains in the corners were grey.

It was cold and uninspiring and he felt conspicuous in his clean blue jeans and blue and yellow rugby shirt. Even Rachel, who'd taken the garden chair, was dressed head to toe in grey, as if her intention was to disappear into her surroundings.

She leaned back and crossed thin, bare legs, the higher leg swinging from the knee in agitation, as she watched Marcus setting up the camera and sound equipment. She was nervous, Alex didn't need his special senses to know that, but he could feel a mix of impatience and curiosity coming from her too.

At a nod from Marcus that he was all set, Virginia moved well away from camera shot and Alex knew it was time to begin.

He wanted Rachel to speak first, and it took an uncomfortably long time, but finally, with a quick sideways glance at Virginia before looking back at him, she said, "So, you're a psychic medium from the telly? I'm sorry, I've never heard of you."

Alex smiled at her candour. "Have you ever seen a medium?"

Rachel shook her head. "Why would I? I don't believe in all that stuff."

"So, why did you agree to see me?"

The look Rachel gave him was keen, penetrating, and she replied that the information Virginia had provided—because of what he'd told her—made her wonder. "The stuff she told me, personal things you could only have got from me or from Flora. It got my attention, so here you are." She shrugged her narrow shoulders, her eyes sliding to a scattering of burn holes in the carpet at her feet. "Anyway, what the hell have I got to lose? Things can't possibly get any worse for me, can they?"

"Let me ask you this, Rachel." He waited until he was sure of her attention. "Even if the worst thing should happen following the investigation—and no-one should be under any illusion that I can help you there—wouldn't it at least help you to know what actually happened that day, even if the police couldn't be convinced?"

He could see how she flinched at the mention of the police. Virginia had told him how Rachel had seen the image of Flora's face on an old newspaper and had called the number given. They'd taken samples from her to check against DNA taken from Flora's remains and then the interrogations had begun, for they wanted to know why Flora hadn't been in school, why she'd hadn't seen a doctor or dentist and why she hadn't reported Flora missing six years earlier.

Her reasoning that she would hardly have come forward now if she'd anything to do with Flora's death seemed to fall on deaf ears, but she thought it only a matter of time before she was arrested and charged.

"Rachel, Flora is fine, absolutely fine, she just needs to tell you what happened, and she needs to know in return why you didn't go back. She loves you very, very much but she's confused. You can share the information through me, and then you can both rest easy."

As if she'd been prodded, Rachel suddenly leapt up, looking wildly around her as if she wanted to bolt from the room, but then she apologised and collapsed back into the chair as if she had been drained of strength.

Virginia told her to try and relax and that she'd explained to Alex about the panic attacks. "You can stop the interview at any time."

Rachel nodded and addressed Alex. "I'm sorry. I'm always on edge. Wired, you know? It's been so hard. All these years of wondering, and then when I heard about you—well, truth is, I've been longing for this day ever since, for you to come and tell me, even though I don't really believe you can." She pinched the bridge of her nose. "Six years of not knowing! Can you really see her?"

"Yes. She's here now, beside you. She's been visiting me often since I met her where she died. She's a delightful little girl."

Unlike most people, Rachel did not look around. She didn't believe him, at least not yet, so why make a wasted effort?

Alex described Flora as he saw her, then said, "But you know that her image, the clay model of her face, has been in all the newspapers and on the TV news and I have seen it so I can't offer that as evidence. But I know they didn't get her hair and eye colour quite right, they had to make assumptions about those."

Rachel, her voice a mere whisper, said, "When I first saw the photograph in a newspaper I almost fainted. To see her face again! Yes, some things weren't accurate, but they wouldn't know it all from a pile of bones, would they? How on earth were they able to make that model of her face though, so life-like?"

"I've seen how it's done, it is amazing. But of course, you could say I was guessing the colour of Flora's hair and eyes by looking at you. I need to provide you with proof that I'm communicating directly with Flora, it's vital if this is to work for you. What exactly was it that Virginia told you that made you agree to this meeting?"

Rachel glanced at Virginia then gave a long, slow blink before looking back at him. He sensed that she'd like to light a cigarette, but Flora told him she'd given up because she had a bad chest and they were too expensive. Alex relayed this and Rachel nodded her head, picking at fingernails that were bitten to the quick.

"It was the torch, really. I've never told anyone about that, so I wondered how the hell you could know about it."

"Yes, the torch. Flora told me it was precious to her because she hated the dark and she carried it everywhere. It stopped working and you promised to get new batteries for it, that morning you left."

Rachel's front teeth, one of them with a corner chipped off, bit down on her lower lip and she nodded again with a quick dip of her head.

Alex opened his psychic senses wider and asked silently for Flora to give him more information, more evidence, that he could relay to her mother, telling her how important it was. He listened and spoke at the same time, his eyes closed to concentrate.

"A grey cat. Pink fluffy slippers. You had to leave the slippers behind and she was cross about that. Hemp? She's saying hemp, though I don't know what that means. A mattress . . . it's spread with clothes, yours and hers. You slept on them, but she packed them away while she waited for you. She says you always used to kiss the tip of her nose, you called her Munchkin and that you liked to say hallelujah when things were going well. You said it when you broke into that house, because it was much easier than you'd expected. She's showing me a birthday cake, with pink icing. She was so pleased with you that day because you bought it for her rather than stole it. You both ate it all in one go. She likes pink, she says, because for a while you made her dress like a boy so the bad men wouldn't notice her."

Flinching, Rachel put her hand up. "Enough! Is she still near me?"

"Yes. She's stroking your right hand. Close your eyes and concentrate. Really concentrate. She says to turn your hand over and remember how, when she was really little, you used to trace a circle in the palm of her hand while you said a rhyme that ended in a tickle under her arm. She wants to do that to you. Maybe you'll feel a tingle in your hand and up your arm; that's her energy making contact with you. She's so happy to see you."

Turning her hand so it was palm upwards, Rachel closed her eyes and tears immediately pooled beneath her lashes. She let them fall. She spoke so quietly Alex had to strain to hear her say that she thought she could feel something, like the stroke of a feather, in the centre of her palm, but she was so desperate she couldn't be sure. Alex almost had to look away from the naked anguish in her face.

"Did she... did she suffer? Oh my God, I just didn't know what had happened to her! I got back and she wasn't there, just this pool of blood by the fireplace. I couldn't find her, I thought she'd been taken and I couldn't bear it!"

Her last words ended in a wail and Alex went to her, gathered her in his arms, ignoring the stale smell wafting from her skin, her hair and her clothes.

"She didn't suffer, Rachel, I promise you. I know it's what people always say, but she insists she felt nothing more than a short, sharp pain as she fell and hit her head on the corner of the hearth. It was an accident, a tragic accident. The man didn't mean to hurt her."

Rachel pulled away, apologising. She pulled a tissue from her sleeve and wiped her eyes, blew her nose.

"The police believe she was murdered and I can't convince them I didn't do it. I would never have harmed my little girl, I protected her!"

Waiting until she'd calmed down, Alex returned to the couch with a quick nod first to Marcus and then to Virginia, who was sitting on the equipment case. Alex didn't know where she'd worked before joining Eselmont, but this kind of interview was very likely new to her. Marcus, who'd filmed things far worse than this show of raw, desperate emotion, showed no expression as he concentrated on filming the exchange.

"I know, Rachel, but I'm sure you understand why they'd think as they do. I have no hope of convincing them otherwise, but I felt it important to tell you in person that I know they're wrong. They can only work with hard evidence, something I cannot provide, so as far as they're concerned, because Flora died from a blow to the back of her head and was buried in a shallow grave, she must have been murdered and you are the most likely candidate. But Rachel, Flora tells me it isn't so. You weren't there, and she says you would never have harmed her, not in a squillion years." He paused as Rachel gasped.

"She always used that word," she whispered. "Squillion. Anything bigger than she could understand wouldn't be a million or a billion, it would be a squillion. My God. So, what did happen to my baby?"

Alex described those last moments just as Flora had described them to him, how she'd heard noises and come downstairs, thinking Rachel had returned with some breakfast, but instead there was a man with a scarred face and she'd tried to run past him but his huge body had filled the doorway and she'd run straight into his stomach, winding him.

"The man was as scared as she was, and he shoved her away from him in a reflex action. She fell backwards, hitting her head on the hearth so hard it cracked her skull. He tried to help her, to save her, but there was nothing he could do. He panicked. He didn't want to leave her so he wrapped her in his sleeping bag and buried her, crying and begging her forgiveness as he did so."

"Does she know him? Will he be caught? Because unless he is I don't have much hope, do I?"

Alex couldn't answer whether or not the man would be caught, but he rather thought the police wouldn't even bother looking on the say so of a psychic medium.

"Why didn't you report her missing, Rachel? If you'd done so at the time there would still have been evidence in the house."

She sighed. "I was afraid. I'm the type they don't like to put themselves out for, a shoplifter and a prostitute, a down and out with no fixed address, who'd dragged her little daughter in and out of the worst kind of places. I knew I'd get into trouble for that. Child neglect, they call it. I didn't neglect my Flora! But I didn't know what had happened! What could I have told them? I was in such a state, so scared, I just wasn't thinking straight."

Alex, keeping to himself that his idea of what constituted child neglect was markedly different to Rachel's, replied, "I know, and I'm sorry. But I don't see how the man can ever be located. That entire row of houses was destroyed before her body was discovered and any chance of finding fingerprints or DNA in the fabric of the sleeping bag or the scraps of Flora's clothing was lost after years in the earth. There's the remotest chance that he'll see the publicity and come forward, but I really think the chances of that are next to zero. Flora says she doesn't want you to go to prison but neither does she want him caught, because the whole thing was an accident and who would believe him, a tramp that looked the way he did, and not quite right in the head? Those are her words, not mine."

"But it would get me off the hook, doesn't she care about that? Oh God, what am I saying? I'd rather an innocent man be punished? I'm sorry. I really don't care if I go to the nick, I deserve it." She indicated the shabby room and cheap furniture with a wave of her hand. "At least I'd be warm and dry and fed three times a day and people wouldn't spit at me in the street. It's why I had to leave Manchester. I thought I'd be anonymous here, but everyone seems to know who I am: the mother who murdered her child. But I didn't do it, I swear I didn't! I could never have hurt my little girl."

"Rachel, Flora has her arms around you. She doesn't want you to cry because she's okay where she is."

But Rachel, leaning forward with her head into her hands, was rocking to and fro and crying as if she'd never be able to stop. Alex stayed where he was, smiling reassurance at Flora who was stroking her mother's hair, deciding it was better to let her cry it out now.

He thought it highly likely that Rachel would end up being charged, and there was absolutely nothing he could do about it, for the type of evidence he could offer would hardly stand up in a court of law. But if she could at least believe the truth, that her little girl hadn't been murdered and that she hadn't suffered, she could surely put her guilt about that part of this tragic story to rest.

But prison would be far from an easy ride for her, despite the heating and the regular meals she'd made that weak joke about, for as far as her fellow inmates would be concerned she would be the worst kind of child killer, a mother who had murdered her young daughter and left her to rot in a shallow grave. They would make her suffer for that in all sorts of ways, far more devious and nastier than spitting in her face.

Alex despaired for her, but he knew beyond a shadow of a doubt that he could do nothing to help her if—when—she was arrested.

But, Flora reminded him, there was still more that needed to be said.

"Rachel? Flora's job is done now. She's waited all these years to tell you what happened, now she wants to know what happened to you. Why were you gone so long?"

At Rachel's howl of despair, Alex assured her that Flora held nothing against her, she simply wanted to know because she'd been so worried for her.

"She was worried for me? Oh God! Flora, Flora! I'm so sorry!"

She steadied herself, and Alex could feel her resolve strengthening. He agreed with Flora that her mother needed to tell her part of the story, so Flora could finally go on in peace, so he wasn't going to leave this sad, dingy little flat until it was all out in the open.

Rachel took a shuddering breath and started her explanation, speaking in a low monotone as she relived that day.

"It was pouring. I mean, pouring so hard you couldn't see a yard in front of you. The streets were practically flooded and I only had light shoes on and my coat was soon soaked through. I walked a long way with no sign of any shops and thought I must've picked the wrong direction. I walked up street after street until I could hear cars passing up ahead, and I found a small high street. I had some money and bought a few things in the first grocery store I came to. The batteries were too expensive but I couldn't risk nicking them in case I got caught and couldn't get back to Flora. The bloody irony of that, eh?"

Her voice dropped to a whisper. "It was still pouring when I started to head back, and I got lost! I hadn't been able to keep my bearings because of the rain, so I just didn't know the way back. I don't know how many wrong turns I must've made. I was so cold my teeth were chattering, and I was in a panic, which just made things worse. I didn't even know the name of the street where I'd left Flora so I couldn't ask anyone, even if there'd been anyone out in that weather to ask. I walked and walked, going up and down streets and roads, so desperate but unable to find where Flora was waiting."

Eyes closed, she stopped speaking for a little while. Alex glanced at Marcus and Virginia, signalling that the story wasn't finished yet and they should keep quiet.

Rachel took a breath. "Finally, I recognised where I was; I was close. I ran the rest of the way, climbed through the window and pounded up the stairs. Flora wasn't there, but she'd packed all our clothes in the plastic bags, and there was an empty water bottle and biscuit wrapper on the floor." Rachel swallowed hard. "I ran all over the house calling her name. The front room downstairs was quite dark because of the boarded-up windows, but there was enough daylight to . . . to see a dark stain round the hearth. I . . . I touched it. There was nothing else in that room, just that horrible pool of blood, and I didn't know if was hers, but she wasn't in the house, so . . ."

Alex stopped her. Flora was getting distraught and Rachel, who'd gone alarmingly white, was clearly bordering on exhaustion.

"Let me get you a drink," Virginia said. "Water? Or do you need something stronger?"

Rachel gave a quick smile, a mere twitch of her pale lips. "Brandy please, if there's any left. Over there." She nodded to the small cabinet and Virginia quickly poured what was in the bottle, having to drain it to get a mere inch in the glass.

"Here. Take a sip. This is hard for you, I know, but getting it all out in the open will be cathartic, both for you and for Flora." Alex waited a beat while Rachel drank it down in one swallow. "Flora says she doesn't need to know any more. It's enough that you hadn't been hurt, because that's what she'd been worried about, that you'd been in an accident or something. She's so happy that wasn't the case."

The brandy restored some colour to Rachel's cheeks and lips, and Alex was relieved that their session had indeed been cathartic, for he could feel a marked difference in both mother and daughter. She and Flora both knew all the facts about each other now on that dreadful day, and they could go on from here without being shadowed by the appalling doubts that had hung over them for six years.

But Rachel wasn't quite finished.

"I ran. I ran through every inch of that house screaming for her, then I grabbed our things and bolted, thinking my heart would break. The garden was muddy, I remember that, but you couldn't see very far and I didn't notice anything. I mean, I still couldn't see much because of that bloody rain! If not for that I might have seen—he might have still been there! But I had no idea, how could I? I searched everywhere for her, even went back to Hemp and asked him if he'd taken her to spite me for leaving him. All I got for that was a black eye for taking some money from him and running away. When I realised I had no hope of finding her, and that she was likely dead anyway, I walked and walked until I came to a railway line."

She stopped a moment, turning the empty glass between the palms of her hands. "I thought of ending it. How could I go on without my Flora? Especially not knowing what had happened to her! God knows I hadn't given her the life she deserved, but I loved her! Oh, how I loved her. She meant everything to me. I felt bad about the way things were going for us, but I couldn't stand the idea of her being taken into care, because that was what would have happened if I'd gone to social services."

She swallowed and her voice dropped. "But if I had, she'd be alive, wouldn't she? So, I wanted to die, I really did. But then I thought, what if she wasn't dead? What if she'd been taken somewhere and one day she'd get away and come looking for me? I had to stay alive." Rachel squeezed her eyes shut, reliving every painful second, and the glass tumbled from her hands. "Oh, Flora, my sweet little Munchkin, I'm so sorry! I wanted to keep you safe and I failed. I hope you can forgive me. I don't care what happens to me now, it's enough that I know the truth and that you are happy where you are."

Alex grinned as Flora managed to lift a strand of her mother's hair away from her scalp so that Rachel could feel it. Marcus and Virginia both gasped as they watched it happen.

"Is that her?" whispered Rachel. "Is Flora playing with my hair?"

Alex nodded and in a moment Rachel was on her knees crawling across the carpet to him. She wrapped her arms around his legs, saying over and over, "Thank God for you, Alex. Oh! Thank God for you!"

***

"Wow, Alex, that's really powerful stuff!"

There was a long silence, the atmosphere in the Eselmont conference room electric following the first viewing of the as yet unedited version of Alex's interview with Rachel. Everyone was stunned by the raw emotion captured in the footage. Alex let out a breath and leaned forward, his hands palms down on the table.

"I want that last bit cut. No-one should see her crawling to me on her knees like that. She hasn't been formally charged yet, and she's lucky not to be under arrest, but it's surely only a matter of time. The situation for her is really serious; at worst she'll be charged with murder and at best it will be child neglect and not reporting her daughter missing. It pains me deeply to know the truth of what happened and yet be unable to do anything about it." He put one hand to his chest. "I would willingly go to the court and speak up for her, but no-one there would take my evidence. If ever there should come a day when mediums like me are one hundred per cent believed and can take the stand in a criminal case, I shall be long gone."

Virginia was the first to speak. "It's an incredible interview. I knew it would be as I sat there next to Marcus and watched it unfold. I know you're concerned that you can't prove anything, Alex, but your audience will see it and the media will run with it, and the public will have the chance to make up their own minds. After all, the chance to tell her side of the story is what Rachel wants and she's signed the authorisation to go ahead, no matter what happens to her. Seems to me she doesn't *care* what happens to her."

A gravelly voice spoke up then, and all heads turned towards the Creative Director. Strangely for one working for a production house that specialised in all things paranormal, Nathan declared himself a 'devout sceptic' and 'the voice of reason' in an otherwise crazy company. Everyone absolutely loved Nathan, knowing that he was really only playing devil's advocate for the fun of it; he was as firm a believer as the rest of them, he just wouldn't admit it.

"Most of you weirdos believe in Alex's psychic skills." He

winked at Alex. "But can you imagine how the press are going to react if, and let's face it, it's more likely to be when Rachel is locked up for the murder of her daughter? Alex's credibility could be shot down in flames."

Marcus gave a snort of exasperation. "Alex was able to give the girl's name and lots of personal details about her long before Rachel came forward."

"That's as maybe, but we can't substantiate anything," declared Nathan. "Alex, you can't prove that what Flora told you is the truth, can you?"

There was a collective intake of breath at that and everyone waited for Marcus to explain.

"For the sake of argument, how do we know she's not lying to protect her mother?" Nathan held his hand up to forestall any interruptions and turned to Alex. "Set aside your own emotions for a moment. Isn't what I've just said feasible, that the girl would want to protect her mother? It could well have been an accident as she says it was, but it could have been Rachel that did it, not some tramp. None of the stuff Flora says belonged to that man were left behind, so there's not a trace of anyone else ever being there. Rachel did herself no favours by living the way she did and by not going to the police straight away when Flora went missing. Even when they created an image of Flora's face and plastered it all over the media she still took her time coming forward."

He held up his hand again as objections were raised by Virginia and Marcus. "I know she told you it was because she doesn't read the papers or watch the news, but try convincing the general public of that. No, she might well be a nice girl who fell on hard times through no fault of her own, but I don't think she did right by her daughter, dragging her from pillar to post, keeping her from an education and healthcare, and that's what everyone is going to home in on."

Alex admitted that he had thought of the possibility that Flora might be lying about the big, scarred man, and so had been very careful in his questioning of her. When people lied they usually found it difficult to keep to the details and something seemingly insignificant often gave them away, but Flora's story never wavered, even when he eventually challenged her outright. At no time did his senses pick up anything of deceit or guile from her or Rachel, and he wholeheartedly believed that Rachel hadn't had anything to do with Flora's death.

Nathan continued, "As I said, the media could have a field day with this. Aren't they already sniffing around?"

"I'm not bothered by the media," Alex replied. "Some continue to vilify me since the show first aired and there were a few journalists who were downright cruel when Amber died. Well, I'm still standing!" He paused. "A little girl died in miserable and suspicious circumstances, her mother is very likely going to be found guilty of killing her even though she didn't. For the sake of common humanity we owe it to both of them to broadcast their story with honesty and integrity and allow people to make up their own minds."

There was a "hear, hear" from Virginia and Marcus and a couple of others seated at the conference table.

At last Paul, who hadn't said a word throughout the whole meeting, spoke up.

"We've been contacted by a couple of journos," he said. "I suspect someone from the construction site talked despite our telling them of the need to keep a lid on things until the job was finished. But you can't blame them because it's an intriguing story in itself, and here we are adding to it by giving it a paranormal twist. I suggest we issue a statement along the lines of being sensitive to the case and not wishing to interfere with an ongoing police investigation. Let's divert their interest to the investigation itself and keep referring them to the detective in charge. Heaven knows, there's enough juice there to keep them busy."

There was a murmur of agreement, except from Nathan, who tutted and shook his head.

"A paranormal twist," he said. "Yep, that's what we do, folks!"

Matt, who'd not joined in the exchange, despite having plenty to say before they'd watched the interview, slapped the table, his signal that the meeting was concluded.

"Right, let's get that press statement prepared, and I'd also like some blurb to start and end the programme when it's broadcast. I was thinking to slot it in with one of the programmes like we're doing with the one-to-ones but now I've seen this I think it deserves to stand alone. You all know the kind of thing that's needed. In the meantime, we need to get to work in the editing suite. It's a brilliant interview, Alex, brilliant."

Chapter 20

"Kathleen, I'd like to take a bath by myself. I think if you put a plastic bag on my arm and tape it in place so there's no danger of getting it wet I'll be able to manage."

Gritting her teeth at her mother's insistence on calling her Kathleen, Kallie quickly ran through the logistics of what her mother was asking.

"Are you sure that's a good idea? Well, let me find Gran's rubber mat to make sure you don't slip. I think it's still in the airing cupboard."

"I do not require a rubber mat; those things are horrible to sit on. I'll be extra careful getting in and out. I know you don't enjoy bathing me any more than I enjoy you having to do it, and I most certainly don't want to be continually treated as if I'm an invalid. I'm sure I'll be fine."

Having no choice but to agree, and relieved to not have to see her mother totally naked again, Kallie got the bath ready and put a nice thick towel within easy reach, then returned to the kitchen to hunt down a plastic bag. She didn't have any of the thin plastic supermarket bags that would have been ideal so her mother suggested they try cling wrap.

Kallie used large sticking plasters round the top of Celia's arm above the plaster cast then wound the wrap all the way down and totally enclosed the hand so it stuck to itself and formed a good seal. Celia winced a bit as it went round her fingers, and Kallie did too because they were still sore.

"Okay? I'll leave you to it then. I'll make a start on dinner so just shout if you need me."

Celia went into the bathroom and shut the door and Kallie waited until she heard the splash of water as her mother climbed into the bath. Wearily, she started to peel some potatoes. She hadn't slept well since Celia had arrived because she was too aware of her sleeping in Walter and Verity's bed across the landing. Their meals together were difficult, and not because her mother couldn't manage to eat, because she'd proved quite deft at forking up whatever Kallie served, but because they found it so damned hard to talk to each other. It was a relief for them both to leave the table and sit in front of the television until Celia announced she was tired and going to bed.

With the potatoes coming to the boil, Kallie lowered the heat and tapped on the bathroom door.

"Are you okay, Mum? Do you need any help getting out?"

Celia replied that she was already out and coping just fine and it wasn't long before she came into the kitchen, dressed in her nightie and dressing gown. Her hair had curled in the steam.

"Would you tie the belt for me please? That's the only thing I can't do."

Kallie did so and said, "Wow, I can't believe how much you've managed to do by yourself! How on earth did you get your nightie on?"

"I told you I could manage. Could we eat soon so I can have an early night?"

Kallie agreed, secretly delighted that she would have the evening to herself. Tomorrow she had a full day at the salon and then it would be Sunday. Oh gosh, what would they do on Sunday? Shrugging it off, reminding herself that she had to carry on taking it just one day at a time.

Kallie quickly got their dinner served up. As soon as she'd finished the mashed potato, vegetables and roast chicken, which Kallie had cut up into bite size pieces, Celia said she was going upstairs and would read until she fell asleep.

"Okay. I need to be at work early tomorrow, so shall I help you get dressed before I go?"

"There's no need." Celia indicated her nightwear. "I'm sure I can dress myself from now on. I've been independent all my life, Kathleen, so if I can at least be trusted to do that I think it'll suit both of us, don't you? I don't think you need to leave me breakfast or lunch, either, though I appreciate that you have always thought to do so."

Kallie wanted to dance a jig round the room now that getting Celia bathed and dressed had come to an end, and not just for her sake, of course she was well aware how humiliated Celia felt at having to be helped this way.

Every morning so far Kallie had got up extra early to make her mother some breakfast and a lunch that would be easy for her to manage and then she'd helped her get dressed. The embarrassment they had both felt would always be painful to recall. After the first time, Celia had insisted on putting on her skirt by herself for modesty's sake before Kallie came into the room, but Kallie had still to put Celia's knickers on.

Celia, almost in tears, had said that she would do without tights and a bra, so Kallie had very carefully eased her blouse on, starting with Celia's bad arm, keeping her eyes averted from her bare breasts, and finally draped a cardigan over her shoulders.

Once assured that her mother had everything she needed and would be fine on her own with her books, Kallie happily escaped to the salon where she could immerse herself in aromatherapy oils and beauty products as she made her clients feel good and relaxed.

Unfortunately, it didn't make herself feel good and relaxed, for she dreaded going home. She'd got so used to coming in, switching on the TV, getting changed into jeans and taking it easy with a mug of tea or coffee. Now Celia was there and her routine had had to change quite drastically to accommodate her.

She would be able to escape to the salon tomorrow without even seeing her mother. Kallie said goodnight and promised to keep the television volume down low so she wouldn't disturb her.

"It won't disturb me. I prefer noise to silence, that's why I live on a busy road."

Once she'd gone Kallie decided to watch a sitcom she'd been missing because Celia didn't like it, keeping the volume low no matter what her mother said about not minding noise; the monotonous sweep of passing traffic was quite different to the lively sound of a television.

An hour passed and Kallie contemplated making some hot chocolate, wondering if she should pop up and see if Celia wanted some. Suddenly, though, as if she'd somehow caused her to materialise, there was Celia about halfway down the stairs. Barefoot, in her long white nightdress and with her wild grey hair she looked quite ghost-like and Kallie wondered for a horrified moment if she was sleep walking.

She called out, "Mum? Are you okay? Do you need something?"

Celia came all the way down. "I was asleep. Something woke me."

"Oh, sorry, it must be the TV, though I've got it down really low."

"No. Someone spoke to me, called my name. I thought it must be you."

Kallie shook her head and said her mother must have been dreaming.

"I haven't called you. You're still on strong painkillers, and you said you were really tired. I was about to make some hot chocolate; would you like some?"

Celia smiled then, a smile that reached her eyes and softened her face, and she said she would love some hot chocolate as long as Kallie wouldn't mind if she stayed down with her to drink it. Hiding her surprise, Kallie agreed and went to make it.

When she came back, her mother was sitting on the couch, her legs tucked up under her, her plastered arm resting on her lap.

"You must be cold. Let me get you a blanket."

"Thank you, Kallie, that's very kind."

Kallie! Her mother had called her Kallie! She thought it could very well be the first time that word had ever passed her mother's lips. She fetched a blanket and arranged it over Celia, ensuring her feet were covered. She switched off the television, thinking they might have a go at conversation as her mother was being uncharacteristically sweet.

Celia turned out to be very entertaining and witty, regaling Kallie with some of the student exploits and pranks she'd witnessed over her many years of working at the university.

Watching and listening to this woman sitting across from her and making her laugh Kallie wanted to say, "Okay who are you, and what have you done with my mother?" Of course, she didn't. She didn't dare say or do anything that might spoil the mood. It was so nice!

When they'd drunk the hot chocolate Kallie hoped that their companionable evening would continue, but Celia's face suddenly went quite blank and she looked around her as if not quite knowing where she was. Announcing she should be in bed, Celia got up abruptly, letting the blanket drop to the floor in a heap and she was gone, leaving Kallie wondering what the hell had just happened.

"Well that was surreal," she muttered to herself as she washed up the mugs and the milk pan. It was gone eleven o'clock, far later than she'd intended to stay up, so she went to bed too, setting the alarm for seven the next morning.

Only a few more weeks, she said to herself, as she'd said a hundred times already. *I've just got to get through a few more weeks and then we can go back to our separate lives and our irregular, five-minute phone calls.*

* * *

Feeling like living with her mother for the past four and a half weeks had aged her a good ten years, Kallie called up the stairs, "Okay, that's the suitcase in the car, are you all set?"

Celia's stitches had been removed and the plaster cast had been replaced with a lightweight, waterproof fibreglass one. Once she had found that she could look after herself in every way without difficulty, Celia was determined to go home. Kallie wasn't sorry.

Okay, there had been moments of fun, but most of the time it had been no fun at all with some truly awful arguments, and Kallie feeling constantly wrong-footed by Celia's rapidly changing moods. She was looking forward to having the cottage all to herself again, and to seeing Rosa and her other friends who she'd had to neglect rather than leave Celia in the evenings, as well as the daytimes.

Kallie wasn't yet sure which Celia she would be dealing with today, the mother she was most familiar with, the one who heard voices in the night, or the one who was a funny, kind and caring woman.

There had been no repeats of the phone calls, or the landing light going on and off, or the television playing up, but Celia had insisted on a couple of occasions that the cottage was haunted and Kallie should get the vicar in to exorcise it.

The second time she'd said this, Kallie had asked, "What if it's Gran and Grandad? After all, it's their cottage and they're probably very excited that we're here together."

For a long moment Celia hadn't reacted at all, then she'd exploded, telling Kallie that she was ridiculous and childish if she thought for a second that ghosts existed. Kallie had heatedly retorted that if her mother was talking exorcisms then she must surely believe in ghosts herself, and her mother had amazed her by denying she'd ever suggested such a thing.

Kallie wasn't sure what she believed, but her mother's attitude rankled so much Kallie declared that she positively did believe in life after death, that Verity and Walter were around and Celia would do well to poke her nose out from her rarefied world of laboratories and lecture halls now and then to see beyond the obvious. That had led to yet another of their fierce rows, which ended with the two of them not speaking for a whole day.

Celia appeared, a warm smile on her face.

"I'm looking forward to being back in my own home, as I'm sure you're looking forward to having the cottage to yourself again, but we've had some fun, haven't we?"

Ah, so it was the kind and caring Celia today, the one who called her by her chosen name with friendliness in her voice rather than 'Kathleen' spoken in her usual imperious way.

They got in the car, Kallie keyed in the directions, and they set off on the three-hour journey to Cambridge. Celia kept up a running commentary all the way to their stopping point for coffee, pointing out landmarks and talking more about her university life, and Kallie let her ramble on because it was pleasant to hear Celia talk this way. Besides, she was learning things about her mother, good things, and appreciating how smart she must be to have risen as high as she did in her field. She'd be retiring soon, though, and Kallie wondered how her mother would pass the time when she no longer had her beloved university to go to.

Kallie ordered a cappuccino for herself and a latte for her mother. Studying the pastries, cakes and cookies on display Kallie said, "Mum, do you want anything to eat?"

There was no reply and Kallie turned to find her mother wasn't behind her in the queue. The young man who was there said, "Your mother went off that way, to the shop I think."

"Oh, thank you."

Kallie bought two Danish pastries and carried the tray to an empty table. The shop was opposite but she couldn't see Celia; she must have gone to the toilet. Minutes went by and Kallie was starting to get worried, but at last Celia was heading towards her.

"Gosh, Mum, where have you been? You disappeared without a word and you've been gone ages."

"Can't I go to the toilet without being interrogated?" There was no humour in her voice, no sparkle in her eye.

Uh-oh, thought Kallie. *Nice taken-over-by-an-alien Celia has left the building and horrid mother Celia has returned.*

"Okay, sorry. I hope your coffee's still hot. I got you an apricot Danish."

Celia took a seat and ate the pastry as if she hadn't eaten for a week then drank the lukewarm coffee in a couple of noisy gulps.

"Can we go now? I don't like it here and I want to get home."

She marched off without waiting for a reply.

Kallie, with a sharp exhale, picked up her handbag and followed her mother to the car. The rest of the journey was made in silence, with Kallie seriously wondering if her mother was schizophrenic. These weren't just mood changes, they were whole personality changes, and it was most disturbing.

At last, they pulled up in front of Celia's apartment block. Still not speaking as the lift took them up, Celia stepped out as soon as the doors opened, leaving Kallie to follow with her suitcase. The place felt cold and sterile having been unoccupied for so many weeks and Kallie hoped her mother would open a few windows to let in some fresh air, but Celia just stalked in and out of the rooms as if checking everything was still as she'd left it.

"Wouldn't you like me to take you to the supermarket before I go? I'd feel happier knowing you had a full freezer and everything you need for at least a few days."

"I told you I'll be fine. I'll order online and get it delivered. I'm sure you want to get on your way, Kathleen, it's a long drive."

Heavens, so she was being dismissed, just like that! She

decided to have one more try, though at the same time wondering why she was bothering.

"Mum, are you sure about this? I don't like to think of you being on your own with your wrist not fully healed yet."

"Kathleen, I have been alone all my life. It's the way I like it. I can manage just fine with this new cast, and as you haven't worried about me before I do not understand why you feel you must do so now."

"What? How can you speak to me like that? I—"

Celia put her hand up to stop Kallie continuing. "I know what you have done for me, and I'm very grateful. I will call you in a day or two just to reassure you. You have your own life to live, Kathleen, and I don't want to be a burden to you."

Verity had said virtually the same thing, about not wanting to be a burden, but she had said it and meant it with love. Her mother just wanted her gone and Kallie thought she would burst with indignation.

How dare her mother say such things, how dare she? But she knew that if she stayed a moment longer she would explode and they would be locked in one of their almighty battles and she didn't want to end their time together with yet another argument.

"Okay. I'll go. But please ring me tomorrow evening, don't leave it for days or weeks. We've spent five weeks together without killing each other, Mum, let's remember that, eh?"

She left quietly, the tears not coming until she was well on her way back to Wiltshire.

At least tomorrow, she kept telling herself, things will be back to normal. Tomorrow I'll be at Rainstones House, I'll see Kevin, and I can start enjoying my life again.

Chapter 21

Sylvia gazed up at the sky, lazily making animals out of the fluffy clouds sailing slowly overhead. Flora, lying beside her and chewing on a piece of grass, was giggling at her suggestions of dragons and unicorns. She was surprised the little girl was still with her, because she had fulfilled her wish and communicated with her mother through Alex, so why hadn't she passed through the gate in that high stone wall to the loved ones who were surely waiting to receive her?

Flora had never mentioned her father, grandparents or great-grandparents but it was only logical that someone would be waiting for her just as, she supposed, her own parents were waiting for her to be ready to go through the gate. She knew that Flora liked talking to Alex, and thought he had become something of a father figure for her, but surely she couldn't stay here for all eternity?

Sylvia had yet to communicate with Alex, and couldn't explain even to herself why she was so reluctant to do so. Perhaps it was because she didn't want to hear anything bad about her family, which was cowardly of her, or maybe she wanted to understand and so be able to explain to him why she saw Simon every now and then, even though it was nothing more than a mere glimpse before he was gone again? Flora always saw Simon too.

"Who's that man?" she'd asked the first time she'd seen him and Sylvia had explained it to her.

"But he's not dead like we are, is he? And he doesn't see us."

Sylvia had confirmed that he was not dead, and she didn't know why they could see him and he couldn't see them, but she was sure they would learn the reason eventually.

"You miss him," Flora had said, and it was a statement not a question. *"I miss my mummy, but I feel much better now I've talked to her. I hope she doesn't have to go to prison."*

Sylvia, now she knew the whole story from Flora and Grace, rather thought that was exactly what Rachel would have to do.

"Look!" shouted Flora, bringing Sylvia back from her private thoughts. *"It's a whale!"*

"So it is. And spouting water too, how clever."

Lying there with this lovely little girl, so young and naïve, she hoped never to be disturbed, wanting nothing more than to be left in peace with the warmth of the sun on her face and that small, trusting hand in hers, and for Simon to be with them. But as her lazy mind formed a poodle out of a cloud directly above her something did disturb her. Something she could not ignore.

She pushed herself into a sitting position and looked around, but she and Flora were alone. There was a faint smell on the breeze and she closed her eyes and inhaled deeply to better analyse it. Someone, somewhere, was having a bonfire.

"Do you smell smoke?" she asked Flora.

Flora lifted her face and sniffed the air. *"Yes,"* she replied, wrinkling her nose.

Feeling an invisible, irresistible pull in a certain direction, maybe the direction of the fire where there might be people, she rose and told Flora to stay while she investigated.

"I don't like being alone," Flora said. *"My mummy left me alone."*

"You're perfectly safe here, you know that sweetheart. It never gets dark and the angels are always nearby. I need to go and check something, but I promise I won't be long and I want you to stay put, okay?"

Flora nodded, feeling reassured, so Sylvia set off through the long grass and wild flowers, not bothering to brush away the seeds that rose up and caught in her clothes and her hair.

As she walked, lightly brushing with her fingers the bright red nodding heads of poppies and marvelling at how the cornflowers reflected the blue of the sky, images of her childhood came to her of joyful times when she'd played with her friends in a country meadow just like this.

It seemed a long walk, and the meadow suddenly came to an abrupt end, as if an invisible line had been drawn along the ground from side to side as far as the eye could see. Her next step would take her onto a familiar, lush, close-cropped lawn. She paused between wild meadow and manicured garden, feeling strangely reluctant to go forward. But why? She knew the garden beyond with its colourful flowerbeds and flowing fountain, she and Flora had explored it and discovered interesting statues placed here and there in the glossy dark green shrubbery. She looked for the life-sized stag, sculpted in bronze and placed as if imperiously eyeing the world from its secret woodland hideaway.

Her mood suddenly lifting, she dashed forward, heading for the stag, but she was stopped in her tracks, literally having to stop dead, long before she reached it. In the mere blink of an eye the wall, the very wall that should be way back behind her, had reappeared just yards in front. All she could see was the solid stone that it was built from, too high to scale, stretching either side as far as the eye could see.

As she had when she'd first encountered it she started running, following the wall first one way and then the other in search of the gate. Where was it? As if the thought invoked its presence she saw it some distance away to her right. By the time she reached it, dismayed even further to find it padlocked, the smell of burning was stronger, more acrid, causing the first pang of anxiety to grip her stomach because it did not smell like a bonfire now.

Grasping the bars with both hands, bewildered that the gate was here, padlocked and blocking her way, she peered through and felt her senses reel even more as she saw Simon a short distance away from her. Expecting him to just disappear as he usually did, she was surprised when he remained there, his back to her.

"Simon?" Her voice was just a croak and she tried again. He did not turn; he couldn't have heard her. She called again, louder, *"Simon! Over here!"*

This time he did look her way, but his arms hung by his sides and his expression didn't change, so she couldn't tell if he'd heard her shouting or if he could see her. She yelled again, jumping up and down and pushing and pulling the gate so the chain rattled, calling his name over and over.

The smell of burning was strong now, choking, terrifying, and she knew it had to have something to do with him, with his being here like this, so different from the times before.

Then, suddenly, he looked directly at her. At first, he didn't register who he was looking at, because she was partially obscured by the vertical bars of the gate, but slowly his face broke into a smile which grew wider and wider in delight. He started to walk forward, then, calling her name, he started to run.

Yet he seemed to get no nearer.

Frustrated, she looked up to see if she could get between the top of the gate and the stone arch above it, but it grew in height even as she stared upwards. Simon would have to open the padlock from his side; he could do it, just as she had. She looked back, ready to tell him what to do, and screamed with shock and frustration.

The smell and crackling sound of things burning and melting in raging flames remained, but her husband was no longer there.

***

"Hi Mum. I'm in the car with Alex, we've just arrived in town ... no, we were going to call in a bit later ... well, maybe he's out? No, no, it's fine. Honestly ... yes, we'll go now. I'll call you when we get there. I'm sure he's fine, Mum. He has to leave the house on his own sometimes, maybe it's a good sign ... okay, bye."

"I take it our shopping expedition must be abandoned then, Beth?"

"Afraid so, at least until later. Do you mind? Poor Mum's about to have a root canal and the dentist happened to mention that Pops has missed two appointments. She called the hospital but he's not there and hasn't been there today. She's left messages on his mobile and the answering machine at home and he hasn't called back, so now she's really worried. He has been acting really odd lately, hasn't he?"

Alex didn't want to answer that, because he had first noticed Simon's strange behaviour some time before Paul and Adele's wedding. He simply said, "Okay, let's go."

He took a side street which would get them back on the main road heading in the direction of Simon's house. None of them were coping well with the loss of Sylvia, so long the linchpin of the family, but poor Simon was really struggling, as was to be expected.

He'd been utterly heartbroken at Sylvia's funeral, so heartbroken he'd been sedated by a doctor afterwards because he was near collapse. He seemed to have aged a great deal in a short space of time, and he was much quieter, more introverted, but he still wouldn't drive and steadfastly refused to stay with Anna and Felix even for a short while. However, if no-one called him regularly, he was soon on the phone to Anna, Paul or Beth, using any pretext he could think of to get them to go to his house and stay awhile to keep him company. This was why Anna was so concerned that he wasn't answering her messages.

They all offered to take him out somewhere, even offered to take him away for a holiday, but they could not prise Simon away from his home and his memories.

Less than twenty minutes after Anna's call, they were driving along Simon's street to be greeted by the chaos of two fire engines, a police car, an ambulance, and a small crowd of people who had gathered for the excitement.

Alex was unable to get close to Simon's house, so parked in the first available space alongside the kerb, wondering whose house was on fire, and if Simon was one of the spectators, which would explain why he hadn't responded to Anna's messages.

Beth got out of the car first, and a large woman in a pink and white floral dress broke from the crowd and ran up to her. One of the fire engines roared past them, leaving the scene.

Alex recognised the woman as Mrs Keene, Simon's long-time next-door neighbour, and hurried to hear what she had to say, because he'd seen with a sinking heart just where the emergency was.

"Beth! Oh Beth, my dear, I'm so glad you're here. Your grandad set the kitchen on fire! I was pegging out the washing when I saw black smoke pouring from the window. I looked over the fence and he was outside, just standing there in the middle of the lawn staring back at the house. He didn't respond to my shouts so I called the fire brigade. I wanted to phone your mother, dear, but I don't have her number and Simon said his mobile was inside and he was in too much of a state to remember. The police have been and gone, luvvie, and I think the fire is out."

Mrs Keene grabbed Beth's arm and started to pull her along. "He's in the ambulance, but he's okay. Some slight burns on his arms and face, but thankfully he got out before he could breathe too much smoke. Come on now, come and talk to this gentleman over here, he'll tell you what happened."

Alex and Beth waited beside Mrs Keene as she explained to the fire officer that Beth was the granddaughter of Mr Savarese, the man whose kitchen had caught fire, and Alex her husband. The officer tucked his filthy, flameproof gloves under his arm and shook their hands, reassuring them that the fire had been extinguished and they were just ensuring there was no chance of it reigniting.

"Is my grandfather okay?" Beth asked, not looking much relieved when he assured her that Simon was a little burned and had inhaled some smoke, just as Mrs Keene had said. She was asked to wait a few minutes as he was being treated in the ambulance, then she could go and see him and talk to the paramedics. It was likely they'd take him to hospital, he said, because they'd want to give him a thorough check over.

"Do you know what caused the fire?" Alex asked.

"From what little Mr Savarese has said so far it looks like a forgotten chip pan, sir. Happens all the time." He looked at Beth. "We found a fire blanket in the drawer under the hob, but I suspect your grandfather panicked and threw water on the flames, which is absolutely the wrong thing to do. The fire quickly took hold and spread, and I'm afraid we've only added to the damage putting the fire out. But insurance will get it sorted, and I think Mr Savarese is more shocked than hurt. Which is lucky, let me tell you, because it was like a fireball in there by the time we arrived, and we were here within minutes of receiving the call from his neighbour."

Sounding dazed, Beth thanked him, then said she really must go to her grandad. The fire officer escorted her to the ambulance, and Alex watched as she was helped into it.

Mrs Keene fixed her friendly gaze on Alex. "Turns out that they're the same crew who attended Sylvia when she'd had the heart attack. They said they were sorry to hear that she hadn't survived it. It's a shame, but it has to be said that poor Simon is not coping at all well. It's only to be expected. He and Sylvia were such a wonderfully close couple, of course the poor lamb's finding it a real struggle on his own. I know how often Anna and Beth pop in. I go round when I can, take him a casserole or a fruit pie, and my Len offers to keep him company, takes him for a drink at the local when he's happy to go. But it's not us he wants, is it? Oh, here comes Beth, dear."

Beth said they'd decided to take Simon to the hospital where his burns and throat could be treated, just as the fire officer had predicted.

"I can go with Pops in the ambulance, Alex. He's not badly hurt, I think, but he is in shock. Could you follow us in the car and come and find us at the hospital?"

Alex hugged her, reeling from the need for them all to go yet again to that hospital.

"Of course. Look, you get off now. I'll just check the house to see the extent of the damage and lock up, and I'll come as soon as I've done that, okay?"

Beth started to go back to the ambulance, and suddenly cried out. "I haven't called Mum!" But as she fumbled for her phone in her bag the paramedic called out that they needed to go.

"You go on. I'll phone your mum and leave a message, because if she's midway through a filling she won't be able to talk to me."

When the ambulance had left, with no siren blaring or blue light flashing, which reassured Alex that it wasn't an emergency situation, his mind raced with what could have happened.

Simon had certainly been getting more and more forgetful, which the family put down to his grief and his age, but Alex knew the absent-mindedness had started well before then. Beth seemed either not to have noticed or she had decided to keep her worries to herself until now, but several times Alex had witnessed Simon become confused, and he had seen on more than a couple of occasions before she died the puzzled and concerned expression on Sylvia's face during some of the episodes.

When Simon had been told they wanted to turn off Sylvia's

life support he'd become so agitated they'd all thought he would have to be sedated for his own sake, and since then those episodes had become more frequent and worse.

Had he put the chip pan on the stove to heat up the oil and then just wandered away, started doing some other task and simply forgotten about it? Was it simply a moment of forgetfulness like everyone suffered from time to time or was something more worrying going on?

He made the call to Anna and left a message assuring her that Simon was okay but to call him back as soon as she could. Within minutes she was on the phone, her speech slurred because of her numbed mouth, and she said she would go straight to the hospital.

"Could you check inside the house, Alex? See if it's safe? Obviously Dad is going to have to come and stay with us, he really won't have a choice now, but he'll want to know his house is okay."

"I'm just about to go in, Anna. I'll let you know the situation when I see you at the hospital later. He's going to be fine and Beth is with him, so take your time and drive carefully, okay?"

Alex had actually begun to think that Anna, Beth and Paul were in denial about the state of Simon's mind. They had always found a reason why he asked questions repetitively, forgot to wash himself, shave, change his clothes. He'd mistaken Beth for Sylvia several times, and cried or become angry when he'd realised the mistake. And every time they had all put it down to grief. Alex had been working up to saying something, to suggesting that they get him to the doctor, and now reprimanded himself for not doing so.

The fire officer broke into his thoughts. "Sir? We've done all we can here, so we'll be leaving shortly. It's safe for you go in the house, but I'd advise you to remove any valuables and make sure the property is secure before you leave. Here's a pamphlet explaining what needs to be done and how, but Mr Savarese needs to get onto his insurance company as soon as he possibly can. It looks worse than it really is, but the kitchen and hall will need a complete refit, and I'm certain they'll insist he's accommodated elsewhere while the work is carried out."

Within minutes it seemed that all the emergency workers had packed up and were gone. Mrs Keene had left to pick up her grandchildren from school, and the other neighbours and spectators had drifted away as the drama had come to an end. Alex stood on the threshold of Simon's house, the acrid smell of burning making his eyes water.

As he walked forward and trod on the doormat just inside the door, there was a slight splash; the whole carpet was sodden. Gingerly, he picked his way to the kitchen and peered in. The sight that greeted his eyes made him draw in a sharp breath with shock. He reminded himself that the fire officer had said it was 'not as bad as it looks', but it still looked really bad.

The walls and ceiling were black and peeling, as were most of the cupboard doors, some of which had warped and blistered. Everything that had been on the counter had charred and melted so they looked like lumps of sooty plasticine, and only the electric kettle was still recognisable, though its flex and plastic base had liquefied and fused together. The window blind was a sopping, charred remnant of fabric. The linoleum floor was awash with filthy, black water, staining and making the edges along the skirting boards curl and lift.

Alex checked the rest of the downstairs rooms and apart from the sodden carpet in the hall could see no damage anywhere else. Upstairs too seemed to be fine; fortunately the fire had been contained in the kitchen, but the acrid smell throughout the house was awful and his throat was getting sore.

He found a spare set of keys and left, locking the door behind him. Grateful to be outside in the fresh air he inhaled deeply. A man with a dainty little lurcher on a red leather lead hesitated at the gate, then came forward.

"Alex, we have met before. I'm Len Keene, from next door. My wife told me that you might still be here."

"And she told me that you've both been looking in on Simon. Thank you for that, I'm sure he really appreciates it," Alex replied.

Len shook his head and something about his expression made Alex's psychic senses twitch. He waited, knowing that Len would eventually say what he'd specifically come round to say.

"Um, look, I don't know if I'm speaking out of turn, but, well, my wife thinks I ought to tell someone in Simon's family now that Sylvia's gone."

His curiosity piqued, and not in a good way, Alex asked him to go ahead and listened with growing concern as Len described the day he'd found Simon sitting in the pub garden, lost and confused.

"We've been neighbours and friends for years, and I just knew something wasn't right. Sylvia said it was high blood pressure medication affecting him, but I distinctly remember Simon boasting that he didn't have any of the usual ailments associated with his age. We know Sylvia got an emergency appointment and took him to the doctor that day," he said. "But not what the outcome was. There've been other things happening too. Sometimes it's as if he doesn't recognise me or the wife. We'd make arrangements to go out and he'd forget. Then, when Sylvia was in the hospital, he had that little accident in the car which he blew up out of all proportion and now this fire. Well, as I say, something just doesn't seem right with him, and hasn't done for a while. He wasn't right before Sylvia died and we think he's worse now. Of course, you might know all this already, maybe Sylvia told Anna or your wife and Simon's getting the help he needs, but if you're all unaware of how bad he is—we thought someone ought to know."

***

By the time Alex reached the hospital Simon had been treated for his burns and was in a ward with side rooms each containing four beds. Anna and Beth were sitting with him, and Beth signalled when she saw Alex that she would come out into the corridor.

"They're keeping him in. What did you find inside the house?"

Alex explained about the damage to the kitchen and hall. "There's no question Simon will have to move in with your mum and dad until it's fixed up. I hope the insurance company will pay out, as it looks as if he left a chip pan unattended and I don't know how they treat things like that. The smoke alarm was working though, so the fire officer told me. How is he?"

"I think Mrs Keene was trying to keep me from panicking when she'd said he was okay, because he clearly isn't. He's sleeping now, but he was asking for you. Come in and sit with us. Mum will be happy to see you too."

Relieved that Simon was resting, because he knew that Simon would immediately ask him as he always did if he had yet made contact with Sylvia, he followed Beth into the ward and said hello first to Anna, whose mouth was still numb and lopsided, and then studied Simon.

His face and neck were reddened as if severely sunburned, his white bushy eyebrows entirely gone, and the bare skin shiny, whether because of burn or some sort of ointment Alex couldn't tell. Both hands were wrapped in something resembling cling film, but the doctor had been able to reassure them that he would heal with minimal scarring.

Beth explained to Alex that Simon had definitely inhaled smoke so would have a sore throat for a day or two, and she'd lost count of how many times she'd heard someone say that he'd been lucky. But how had it happened? Sylvia never deep fried anything, considering it unhealthy, and Anna hadn't known they even possessed a fryer.

A nurse came by and checked the patient treatment file hanging at the bottom of the bed and said, "He'll sleep on and off for a couple of hours, and he won't be up to talking much when he wakes as his throat will be very sore, so why don't you go on home? We have your number, but there's really nothing to worry about. He'll need a couple of days with us, but he'll be feeling a little better after a good long sleep."

Anna wouldn't leave. A little stunned to find themselves in the hospital and sitting at the bedside of a family member yet again, Alex and Beth decided to stay a little while longer to keep her company.

Alex could see that Anna was tired and distressed but she insisted she wasn't in pain; that would come when the injections the dentist had given her had worn off. He would have to find an opportunity to talk to her in private about his conversation with Len Keene, because he was pretty sure that if she knew anything about Simon's mental state she'd said nothing to Beth and there must be a reason for that.

Beth kept up a bright conversation, determined not to cry.

Too many tears had been spent already, she said, and she was reassured to know that her grandfather would be fine once the burns had healed and now he would have to go and stay with Anna and Felix, which could only be a good thing.

Beth said she'd go outside and call Paul, and Alex pounced on the chance to talk to Anna.

"Anna, there's no delicate way of saying this and I haven't said anything to Beth or Paul, but did Sylvia tell you that she had to take Simon to see the doctor?" He related what Len Keene had told him.

Looking shocked and upset, Anna shook her head. "No, Mum never said anything. But we all know something's wrong, don't we Alex? I mean, his strange behaviour can't all be down to grief, can it? Oh dear, I just haven't wanted to face up to it, which is utterly stupid of me. I'm going to have to do something, I just have to think what. I'll talk to Felix tonight. Thank you Alex, I appreciate you telling me, and thank you for not telling Beth or Paul. I'd rather they didn't know until we know, although I'll understand if you're uncomfortable keeping secrets from Beth."

"It's fine, Anna. There's no sense in worrying her or anyone else until you have the facts. How about you talk to the doctors here? Maybe they can check him over with this new knowledge in mind and you can take it from there."

Simon's eyelids fluttered, and he came to with a startled groan.

Anna immediately ordered him not to move. "You're going to be fine, Dad, but you need to keep still and rest. Are you in pain?"

He shook his head slowly from side to side and tried to speak, but his throat was so sore it came out as if he were talking through gravel and they couldn't understand him. Anna held a glass of water to his lips.

"Don't try to speak Dad, just sip some water. Look, Beth and Alex are here too. We'll be leaving shortly because the nurse is already making signals that we should go, but I'll be back tomorrow, okay? You're going to come and stay with me and Felix for a little while until you're better."

Simon fixed his eyes, shiny with unshed tears, first upon Anna, then on Beth.

"Sylvia," he whispered.

The two women glanced worriedly at each other, but Alex felt a shiver go through him. Had the ordeal of the fire robbed Simon of the knowledge that Sylvia was gone? Simon switched his gaze to Alex and he tried to raise his bandaged hand towards him. His lips moved but Alex had to lean forward and put his ear close to Simon's mouth.

He whispered, "I saw her."

Chapter 22

"Are they absolutely sure, Mum? I can't believe it."

"Neither can I darling, but the tests and scans have led to this diagnosis. We all admit now that we knew Dad was in bad shape even before Mum died. We refused for far too long to see it for what it was, but I am assured by the specialist that there was nothing we could have done that would have made any difference to the progress of the disease."

"Alzheimer's." Paul said the word as if it spelled the end of the world.

Alex, his arm around Beth, wasn't participating much in this family council of war, called by Anna after she'd learned Simon's test results yesterday. It had taken time, but eventually Anna had discovered that Simon had missed two hospital appointments that had been made before Sylvia's death. She had had to work hard to get his tests back on track as soon as possible because Simon proved far from co-operative.

Anna, Beth and Paul were naturally the ones most in shock, for the diagnosis, though not entirely unexpected, had rocked them to the core. Felix said they needed to think carefully about Simon's long-term care.

"Oh Felix, he'll stay with us! I will look after him."

"Anna, were you listening to the doctor? The behaviour he's exhibiting now is bad enough, but it will get a lot worse. We need to plan for his going into a care home eventually. The house will definitely have to be sold now."

Alex knew how Simon was going to take that. He was still asleep in the guest room upstairs, having been living with Anna and Felix since his discharge from hospital after the fire. The morning was passing, though, and there was still no sign of Simon coming down. Did he understand what was happening to him? Alex wondered. Quite likely he did, for he still had many lucid moments, and Anna had elected to be honest with him.

There was a lot of heated discussion going on around the kitchen table, and Alex decided it would be wise to keep his counsel while the blood members of the family argued it out, though he agreed with Felix that Simon's home should now be sold to contribute to the eventual care home fees. Insurance had paid out for repair and redecoration but the house had stood empty all this time, and it was obvious that Simon would not be returning to it.

Since the chip pan incident that had started this whole process, Simon was constantly insisting to them all that he regularly saw Sylvia. Alex had pondered long and hard on this, wondering why he couldn't communicate with Sylvia if Simon could. He had tried many times, hoping to learn how she was and to clarify things regarding Simon, but she did not come through and he could only surmise that it was because she didn't want to. His father had vanished with Alistair again, exploring some other distant realms, so he hadn't been able to ask for his help in finding her.

***

Woken by daylight seeping around the heavy curtains Simon presumed it must be time to get up and make Sylvia her mug of morning tea as he always did. He put his hand expecting to encounter her arm or the curve of her hip, but when he encountered nothing but cool sheets he opened his eyes and stared in confusion at the ceiling. It wasn't the ceiling he expected to see.

His ceiling had swirls in the plaster and a pendant light with a fabric shade in the centre, this one was smooth with a light that had three bare, candle-shaped bulbs in brass, upward-curving arms.

Had he overslept? Pushing himself up so he could see the clock, he was further nonplussed to find there was no clock where it should be and no mahogany tallboy the alarm clock should be sitting on. The walls were painted a pale peachy colour, not papered with the blue and cream patterned wallpaper chosen by Sylvia that he had put up himself one rainy Sunday.

Confused, he pushed back the duvet, not recognising its cover either. Sitting up, he swung his legs over the side of the bed and searched with his feet for his slippers, relieved to see that he was wearing familiar pyjamas and his leather slippers were where they should be. He slid his feet into them, but when he stood the momentary comfort he'd felt slipped away and he felt tears of fear and alarm prickle behind his eyes.

He did not know this room.

He did not know why he was in this room and not in his own home. Looking around he realised that he might have been here before, in fact he was becoming more certain of it by the minute, but not being able to recall the rest of the house beyond it made his heart pound, his head hurt.

Thoughts whirled through his befogged brain as he tried to recall getting into bed last night. He could see his clothes, all neatly folded, on a white rocking chair next to a low, white chest of drawers, but could not remember taking them off and placing them there. On top of the chest he could see his wristwatch and his wallet. He could not remember putting them there either. He noticed that there were shiny patches of skin on his hands. Reaching up to his face, he felt the stubble of a beard that must be several days' growth.

"Sylvia?"

Had he said that out loud? Now he was no longer in a bedroom, no longer in a room at all, but in a garden which he knew, yet didn't know. He turned a half circle and found himself facing a high wrought iron gate set in an archway in a stone wall.

So familiar, yet not.

Like a dream. Yet not a dream.

He walked resolutely forward, calling out for Sylvia. He couldn't have said why he knew she was there, he just did. His heart knew, his soul knew that his beloved was near.

"Simon!"

There she was, behind the gate, waiting for him! He closed the distance between them and reached out his hand to take hers. They connected and the world stood still as they gazed at each other, not speaking because they didn't need to. Her happiness spread through him, and his into her until it felt as if the gate simply melted away leaving nothing between them. They were melded as one, enclosed in their own bubble where no harm could touch them.

Safe. Warm.
Together.
"Simon! No!"
At Sylvia's cry the world tilted, tipping him off balance. Sylvia reached out to hold on to him, pleading with him not to leave her again. But he was being pulled backwards now, unable to stop himself from tumbling over and over in the dark until her dear voice was lost to him, replaced by a loud and insistent buzzing in his ears.

With a heavy thud he fell to his hands and knees onto the carpeted floor, then pitched forward so that he was lying flat on his face.

Winded, confused, he rolled over onto his back and lay where he fell, his fingers digging into the short pile of the carpet. Carpet, not grass. That smooth ceiling above his head again, the light fixture coming in and out of focus. Wherever he had been, the place where his Sylvia waited for him, he was not there now.

He hauled himself up and walked slowly to the closed door, trying to orient himself. On a hook on the back of the door hung his faded blue towelling robe and he quickly pulled it on, tying the belt tightly round his waist, welcoming the familiarity of its feel and smell. He put his ear to the door, listening hard for any sounds coming from the house, but he could hear nothing; no voices, no signs of people moving about.

Carefully, he eased the door open and peered out onto a landing. It was thickly carpeted in a different colour to the bedroom. In front of him a white balustrade guarded the staircase. He was in the end bedroom, there was a bathroom to his right and two other doors to his left. At last, he could hear other people downstairs. He went carefully downward, following the voices and the chinking sounds of cutlery on china plates until he was in the kitchen.

The conversation suddenly stopped and several heads swivelled to look at him.

"Dad! You're up! You've slept a long time and missed breakfast, we're all on lunch now. What would you like to eat? Eggs and bacon? Cereal? Toast?"

The woman who had spoken was looking at him expectantly, but her expression changed when he didn't —couldn't—answer her. *Who was she?* Simon thought.

"Dad?" she came towards him, and he stepped back smartly, his hands out as if warding off her approach. "Dad, what's wrong? Did you have a bad night again?"

Simon stared at the upturned face, the hazel eyes framed with rimless glasses looking at him with such concern. He studied the other people in the room, a man and a woman seated at the table, two men, one much older than the other, leaning against the worktop. Who were all these people?

And then he knew. He knew everything. It was as if someone had removed the top of his skull and momentarily removed all memory from his brain, just scooped every single one of them out, and then poured them back in again and closed his skull with a sharp click.

His knees began to buckle but he caught himself and staggered backwards a couple of steps. Felix and Paul rushed forward and sat him down. Simon stared at the people staring back at him and almost laughed with the sheer delight of knowing who they were.

His daughter, Anna, and his son-in-law Felix; Beth and her husband Alex; Paul, his oh-so-successful, entrepreneurial grandson. Paul should get married, he thought. No man should be without a loving wife like his Sylvia was to him and Anna was to Felix. Beth had let the side down a bit by leaving her husband, but she had been so sad after losing the baby. At least the separation hadn't been for long and they were together again now. Yes, he remembered everything and it felt so good.

He asked for scrambled eggs on toast and watched Anna happily bustle about making it for him. He was a lucky, lucky man, with his family surrounding him with such love and his beloved Sylvia waiting for him not far away. Did they know that she was close and he visited her? His eyes rested on Alex. He was a strange one. Simon bet he knew where Sylvia was.

A plate of food was placed in front of him and he picked up a knife and fork. Someone passed him the bottle of ketchup. He ate the eggs with relish and added sugar to the mug of tea placed before him by Beth.

At that moment another woman arrived, calling out a hello as she entered the kitchen. She didn't notice Simon. Paul went to her and kissed her and she nestled into him with her back to Simon as Paul asked, "Was Lily okay? Did you get her plan for the new shop sorted out?"

"Oh yes. Isn't it fantastic that she's confident enough to open another shop?" She pulled away from Paul and held out her hand to Anna. "How's Simon today?" she asked.

Simon slammed down his knife and fork and barked, "And just who the hell are you, young lady?"

Chapter 23

Kallie smoothed out the disposable paper cover on the therapy couch, gave a swift glance around, and told herself she was ready for another busy Thursday in the DPU. There was a light tap on the door. Hmm, were they starting half an hour early today? She called out to the person to come right on in, and Trish popped her head round the door.

"You're wanted in the office, Kallie."

"Pam's office?"

"No, the main one. They're asking if you could pop up there now. It sounded urgent. Let me know when you're back and I'll bring the first guest in."

As Trish's head withdrew, Kallie wondered what on earth anyone in the main office would want with her. Had she done something wrong? She didn't think so, but couldn't help feeling a little nervous as she made her way to the oldest part of the sprawling building where the administrative team worked on the first floor. As she went in, she realised Trish hadn't said who she should ask for, and at least six people were sat at desks working.

"Hi, I'm Kallie Harper. I was asked to come up here?"

"Oh yes, Kallie. It's Sasha who wants to see you, go straight in."

Sasha was Head of Personnel, making Kallie even more worried that this had something to do with her employment there. The door was open, but Sasha was scribbling on a notepad so Kallie knocked to let her know she was there.

"Ah, Kallie. Thanks for coming so quickly, I'm aware you're always busy in the DPU, so I won't keep you long. Have a seat."

Really curious now, Kallie took the chair on the other side of the desk.

Sasha opened a file and selected a typed letter from it. "Kallie, I have been having dealings with your mother's solicitor, under strict instructions not to inform you until a certain event had taken place. It has been a mighty uncomfortable time for me, I want you to know that, for I have not understood the need for such secrecy. However, my hands were tied by legal requirements drawn up by your mother's solicitor and agreed by our own legal advisors. I understand that you and she are virtually estranged, is that right?"

Taken aback by the directness of Sasha's question, Kallie replied, "I wouldn't say estranged. We don't see each other but we do talk on the phone. Not regularly, if I'm honest, but we try very hard to stay in touch." She gave a rueful smile. "I'm afraid we're not very good at it."

"Hmm. Well, Kallie, there's no easy way to say this, so I'll just come straight out with it. Your mother has been diagnosed with vascular dementia, and the event of which I speak is about to take place. She is coming here, as a full-time resident in the dementia care wing."

Kallie could say nothing, only stare. It was too much unbelievable information to absorb in one go. Celia hadn't said a word about her illness and now she was coming here? And she'd planned it all through a solicitor? How the hell had she managed it? If Kallie wasn't sitting down she'd fall down. She felt hysteria gathering somewhere under her ribs and had to fight hard to stop it rising and coming out in a cry of rage from her throat. Why had Celia gone about it this way instead of picking up the damned phone and telling her? Kallie would have helped her. She would have!

"Are you all right, Kallie? Shall I get you some water?"

"No! Um . . . no, thank you. I'll be okay in a minute."

"I understand the shock you must be feeling. If you ever need to talk to someone, you know you can go to any of the counsellors here, don't you?"

Kallie nodded, filing that information away for she might well be in need of counselling after this. Despite hearing what Celia had, a condition she knew nothing about but was in the right place to find out, Kallie felt embarrassed, even betrayed. How must it look to Sasha and anyone else here who knew about this?

After a struggle she found her voice. "When is she coming in?"

"Monday next week. Her room is almost ready and she should arrive about mid-afternoon. Kallie, you're very pale, would you like me to ring Pam and ask her to reschedule anyone booked in to see you today? It would be quite understandable if you'd rather go home."

Tempting though it was to walk out of this office, out of the building, into her car and just keep driving until she ran out of road or fuel, Kallie said she would be fine to continue. In fact she would rather continue, for the guests coming in for their therapies would help to keep everything in perspective.

After Sasha had assured her that her mother had made all the necessary financial arrangements and Kallie needn't worry about a thing as far as Celia's residency at Rainstones House was concerned, Kallie left her and scurried back to the hospice wing and the sanctuary of the DPU, wishing that Kevin was working today. He always cheered her up, and she was beginning to suspect, to hope, that he felt about her the way she was beginning to feel about him. But she was meeting him for drinks tomorrow evening, so that was something to look forward to.

She let Trish know she was back and went to the treatment room to wait for her first guest. She would put all her worries about her mother to the back of her mind for the next few hours so she could concentrate on making people coping so stoically with their life-limiting illnesses feel just a little bit better.

Part Four

THE WAITING GATE
2017

Chapter 24

Alex rubbed the tiredness from his eyes and massaged his temples with small circular movements. He was exhausted. With the Eselmont programme finally being aired after a lot of wrangling between two channels fighting over the rights to broadcast it and the publicity all that entailed now in full swing. His latest book less than three-quarters written with a deadline looming, and poor Simon in Rainstones House sinking further and further into dementia, he felt pulled in too many directions.

Today he had a rare Sunday off. He and Beth were about to go to Rainstones House, but first Alex needed to see his dad and have a little time with Amber to help recharge his batteries.

While Beth was busy elsewhere in the house he went into the living room and settled into his father's wine-red, deep-buttoned leather chair. Leaning his head back and placing his palms on the smooth, worn curve of the arms, he opened his mind and called.

His father was immediately there, with Alex's little girl playing on the floor at his feet.

"Hi Dad. Still having fun with Alistair?"

"Oh aye, he hasn't changed a bit, still loves to adventure and explore, and I'm enjoying making new discoveries with him. He thoroughly enjoyed watching us work together on your show, though, and is wondering if he can be a guide himself. How do you feel about having the two of us helping you out?"

Alex laughed at the thought of having his father's Scottish tones in one ear and his uncle's Scottish-with-an-Aussie twang in the other.

"That would be great, Dad, if you can teach him to be as good as you are!"

"Oh, you need have no concerns there; he's a fast learner. He's off exploring by himself for a wee while. I rather think there's a special lady over here he's trying to find, though he's being un-typically coy about it. I told him to look out for your Sylvia while he's about it, because I haven't been able to make contact with her. Now then, here's your Amber. She's always such a happy little thing."

By the time Beth called that she was ready to go out Alex felt much happier, his energy renewed. He held Beth close as he told her that their little girl was absolutely fine, and by the time they got on the way to the care home, he felt able to cope with anything.

The smell of roast beef and cabbage filled Alex's nose as soon as he and Beth entered the dementia care wing. No need to ask what the residents had had for lunch then. He signed in the visitors' book for them both and trailed Beth into the 1950s-style lounge.

As they got closer, he heard an angry, raised voice and recognised with a sinking heart that it was Simon, a sure sign that this was one of his bad days. When Simon came into view Alex could see that he had a face like thunder. Spraying spittle he was shouting at poor Anna, who looked very small in front of his towering rage as she tried to keep clear of his flailing arms.

"I do not want to spend another minute in this godawful place! Where is Sylvia? Tell her to get here right now, I want to go home!"

Rainstones House was as far from an awful place as you could get, but there were times that Simon did not to know where he was.

Placing him in a care home had been an agonising decision for Anna, Beth and Paul, but one they'd had to take and they'd been so pleased to secure a place for him here.

His descent into the mean grip of dementia had been astonishingly rapid once he'd been fully diagnosed, almost as if the diagnosis itself had caused the acceleration. All too soon after he'd arrived to stay with Anna and Felix because he was no longer capable of living alone, Anna had tearfully admitted that she couldn't cope because his behaviour had worsened to the point he was unpredictable and a danger to himself.

They had all watched in dismay as Simon's memory lapses and mood swings became steadily more severe and frightening. More than once, Anna had discovered that he was missing from the house, and on one of those occasions she'd discovered him outside fumbling with a set of keys, trying to get into her car. Thank goodness he'd been trying to open the door with the wrong key and hadn't thought to use the remote because it made the blood run cold to think what might have happened had he managed to get into the car and drive off.

In between the episodes of manic behaviour, his periods of complete docility were a welcome respite, though still heart breaking because it was as if he was there only in body, his mind having gone a-wandering who knew where. He didn't wash or shave unless he was told to. Sometimes he spent the whole day shuffling about in his pyjamas and slippers.

The final straw for Anna had been the morning he had walked into the kitchen stark naked, just as she was serving coffee and biscuits to some friends, and he'd become aggressive when she'd ordered him to go and put some clothes on.

The temper tantrums had been the worst thing, though, because they were so uncharacteristic and his volcanic eruptions truly frightening. And here he was, throwing another almighty strop at the one person who always seemed to be his main point of attack—Anna.

Beth started to rush forward to support Anna when it looked as if Simon might strike her but Alex gently held her back as Erin, one of the senior nurses they all respected tremendously, went to Simon and simply said something which caused him to calm down, smile at her and go back to his chair.

Erin followed him, grabbing from the bookshelves his life story scrapbook that Anna had put together and gesturing to Anna to come and sit with them. Alex saw how Simon's body relaxed as Erin opened the book and pointed to some photographs, asking questions about them, and he admired the nurse even more as she continued to hold Simon's attention for a few minutes more even though another ruckus was starting in the far side of the room. When she handed the scrapbook to Anna and went to deal with the next crisis after taking the time to say some reassuring words to her, Alex and Beth went over to join them.

Anna was visibly shaken and a little tearful, but Simon had closed his eyes and was resting his head against the high-backed armchair, his body relaxed, his face slackening to blankness.

After a few minutes, when it seemed likely that Simon

would remain quiet and docile as he usually was following a fit of temper, Anna said she needed to go for a walk and get a breath of fresh air.

"Do you mind if I go with Mum?" Beth said to Alex. "We'll only be about five minutes."

He said he was quite happy to sit with Simon for as long as they wanted, and the two women left. Mulling over the scene he'd just witnessed, Alex wondered how the staff dealt with these outbursts on a daily basis, not to mention the repetitive questions and behaviours. Respite was often short, with the whole thing starting up again, over and over, day in day out. Having mere admiration for the care staff was not nearly enough.

Erin was still attending to the wild-haired woman who'd started shouting abuse while she'd been dealing with Simon. The woman had almost tripped over a walking stick, Alex had no idea if it was her own or someone else's, and Erin was trying to soothe her with her soft voice.

Suddenly, the woman stopped shouting and set off round the perimeter of the room, not seeming to focus on anything yet walking at a cracking pace. Alex watched her, bemused that though she was moving with apparent purpose she looked as expressionless as Simon.

A young woman in jeans and pale blue sweater picked up the abandoned walking stick and placed it where it wouldn't be a danger to anyone, then she waited, watching helplessly as Erin called a young nurse to help and they gently steered the fast pacing woman out of the lounge. Compelled to speak to her, Alex checked Simon to make sure he was still in his own world, then he went over to introduce himself.

"Hello. That was distressing for you, is there anything I

can do? My name's Alex, and that's my wife's grandfather over there."

She gave him a tired smile. "I'm Kallie. That was my mother. I heard your wife's grandfather shouting before my mum started up. Awful, isn't it, seeing them this way? I didn't even know my mother knew so many swear words!"

Alex suggested that they sit down, placing himself so he had a clear view of Simon in case he came out of his trance-like state.

"Has she been here long?"

Kallie sighed and told Alex that it had been almost eighteen months. "She lived in Cambridge, but when she was diagnosed she made arrangements to come here so she could be near me. The nurses tell me that this purposeful walking is quite common. They don't know why it happens. There are others here just like her, and would you believe they can walk themselves to exhaustion? Apparently, they get fed and given fluids even as they're on the move if needed, because they are so driven and trying to stop or restrain them only makes things worse."

"So where have they taken her?"

"Oh, thankfully this is an enlightened care home and as well as the organised entertainments, the sensory rooms and communal lounges like this one—I just love all the 1950s-style furniture and everything, don't you? There's a special place where they can walk in safety, even go outside if the weather's good and they're determined to go out. Honestly, though, it's weird watching them. They move as if they know where they're going, yet they go round and round in circles and never communicate at all. But who knows what goes on in their heads? Is your wife's grandfather like that?"

Alex heard the question but was distracted before answering

because a man and woman had appeared from thin air behind her. Opening his psychic senses he asked if they had a message for her, but either they deliberately ignored him or he hadn't managed to reach them for they didn't acknowledge him in any way.

Thinking quickly to cover his brief distraction, for Kallie was looking at him curiously, he said, "I'm so sorry, I was absorbing what you just said. No, I don't think Simon does that walking thing; I'd no idea it happened to anyone until you told me. In fact, I'd very little knowledge of dementia at all until Simon was diagnosed. There's such a range of symptoms and outcomes, and everyone's different, it seems. Simon used to go wandering about when he lived with my in-laws but I don't know if he does that here. Most of the time he just seems to disappear inside himself, only coming back now and again to rant about something. We're just glad we have a wonderful place like this practically on our doorstep."

"Yes, it's an amazing place. The staff are so compassionate and caring. I've been to a few of the entertainments and the other week they had a couple of pet therapy dogs come in and the patients were allowed to stroke them. It amazed me how much those dogs lifted the atmosphere as soon as they came in and provoked such positive responses." She paused and sighed. "I was only familiar with the hospice side of this place until my mother came in as a resident. My grandfather died there, and I work there as a holistic therapist one day a week. A friend of mine, a Day Patient Unit volunteer, her father's been here for years and years. Trish told me about it but I never dreamed I'd be visiting anyone in here."

"Trish? Trish Gartner?"

"Yes, that's right. You know her, obviously. Her father's

completely bed-bound and totally unresponsive, isn't that awful?"

At that moment Anna and Beth came back from their walk in the garden, and Alex made the introductions.

"Your mum is a patient here?" asked Beth with sympathy. "Gosh, she must be young."

Kallie smiled. "She's not far off seventy. She was nearly forty when she had me. But dementia can strike any age, even in children, so I understand. Mum's in great health physically, so she could be here for a long time."

Beth asked where Kallie's mother was now and she explained again about the safe room.

"I won't see her again today, because she'll walk herself to exhaustion and they'll put her straight to bed. She was only here a matter of weeks before her memory became severely affected and it wasn't long before she didn't recognise me anymore." Kallie looked rueful. "Sorry, you don't want to hear all that when you're probably going through the same thing. It was nice to meet you, though I'm sure we all wish it was under better circumstances."

Kallie gathered up her coat and bag and left the lounge, giving Alex, Beth and Anna a small smile and a wave of her fingers. Alex followed her with his eyes.

"I know that look," said Beth. "Does she have someone with her?"

"Two people," he replied. "Her grandparents, I think. I could sense them when she and I were talking, but they seemed not to be aware of me. I think they're just watching out for her."

"Maybe Kallie's mum is their daughter and that's why they're here, watching over both of them?" Beth squeezed his hand. "Why don't you go outside for a bit Alex?"

He set off to find his favourite bench, the one hidden from the lounge windows but with a good view of the striking water feature.

Once past the area that had been laid out as a giant checkerboard, Alex was pleased to find there was no-one else around. He sat down and contemplated what he'd just witnessed inside, allowing the gentle, musical sound of running water and the little tinkling copper bells to soothe him. He decided he didn't know nearly enough about dementia in general and Simon's condition in particular, and needed to do some research. If only he had the time! He shouldn't even be here now, but he'd come for Beth's sake and he was glad that he had.

"Would you mind if I sit here?" a friendly voice asked, bringing him out of his reverie. "It's my favourite place as it can't be seen from the house and I can get a precious few minutes uninterrupted."

Alex looked up at the slender figure in front of him, delighted to see that it was Erin, and invited her to join him.

She sat down beside him, her knees audibly clicking. "Sorry about that." She laughed. "My knees have always clicked and the years of bending and lifting takes a terrible toll on the joints, even when you've been trained to do it right. Shame Simon had to go into one of his strops just as you and Beth were walking in. Is Anna okay?"

"She's fine and you were marvellous, as always. It amazes me how you stay so calm. Would you like to be alone? I'd say you deserve some peace and quiet after what you've just had to deal with, but I suppose it's all part and parcel of the working day for you, isn't it?"

He made to rise but Erin placed her hand on his arm and gently but firmly prevented him from leaving.

"Actually, Alex Kelburn, I've been stalking you!" She laughed, making her face look years younger. "I've seen every episode of your TV show, I've read your books, and whenever you've come to the hospice to give one of your inspirational talks I've been sure to be there. Everything about you is absolutely fascinating to me and since your wife's grandfather came in I've been waiting for an opportunity just to talk to you! Can I ask you a question?"

She bit her bottom lip and a slow blush rose from her neck upwards as she waited for his response. He assumed she was going to ask if he could give her a message from a late member of her family or a friend, so he nodded, wanting to be generous to someone who worked as hard and as compassionately as she did.

Everyone noticed how kind, how gentle she always was with the residents, and the dementia lounge seemed a much duller place when she wasn't on shift. She asked her question but it wasn't at all what he expected.

"Where do you think they go, the patients who no longer seem to be aware of themselves or their surroundings? I mean, take Simon. One moment he's angry and shouting, the next it's as if he's simply left his body behind and gone somewhere. Some of the patients are like that all the time, never having lucid moments at all, and I've always wondered . . . where do they go?"

Alex showed his surprise and confusion with raised eyebrows.

She laughed, a little nervously, and flapped her hand at him. "Oh, it's probably a stupid question. They're not dead, are they, so how would you know?"

"It's not stupid at all, Erin. In fact, you've just made me wonder about it myself. As you say, they haven't crossed over, so I don't sense them, but they're not here either, are they? Simon insists that he sees his late wife, and I've never seen her so perhaps there's some place ..." He tailed off, a glimmer of an idea taking form in his mind. "It's a fascinating question, and I'm glad you asked it. I shall give it a great deal of thought and see what I can find out."

"Thank you! Oh, thank you for taking me seriously! You've no idea how many people I've tried to talk to and just been dismissed as being fanciful or mad! I honestly believe they go somewhere, just like we do when we die, and I'd give anything to know where. Maybe it's the same place!" She smiled at that thought. "You know, I overheard you talking to Kallie Harper. Her mother is another case in point, though she exhibits markedly different behaviour to Simon. Mostly, she's what we call non-verbal and non-engaging, but with occasional outbursts of swearing, which Kallie tells me she never did before. Then she has to move and keep moving.

"Many are like that, behaving like they're clockwork toys that've been wound up and set going until they wind down again. We call it sundowning because they usually start late afternoon or early evening. If we try and stop them, as we used to do before care protocols changed, they can become really agitated, sometimes aggressive and they and care staff have actually been injured."

"Have you been hurt?"

"Only once, a cracking right hook to my jaw! I was bruised for days, but you can't get angry about it. They don't know what they're doing." She sighed and shook her head. "It pains me to say it, but when I started out it was accepted practice to restrain them when they got agitated. We had this horrid thing called the Buxton chair, which had a built-in table to prevent them from standing up and wandering away by themselves. It took time to make us realise that restraint could sometimes be more dangerous and increased rather than reduced accidents, but by the time I moved here things were already changing and I'm so glad things are different now.

"Care in specialist homes like this one is so much kinder, I think, because the patient is at the heart of everything we do. We sit with the family and take as full a picture of their relative as possible, and we suggest that they put a scrapbook together that we can hold here, just as we did with Anna and Simon's grandchildren."

"Yes, it's what you used to calm him down just now, isn't it?"

"Exactly. As all the staff have access to these vital little biographies that set out some history and likes and dislikes we have an idea of the patients' family, their past and social lives and so on, and we can use the information to engage with them, or for distraction if we need to. Simple things, like asking them if they want a cup of tea, or giving them some small task to do, it all helps to make life a little easier. Back then we constantly tried to keep them in the present; nowadays we go into their reality and use gentle, persuasive techniques to divert and encourage them in ways that won't stress them."

She paused again, then her hand flew to her mouth. "Oh my goodness, listen to me rabbiting on! You've good ears on you, Alex Kelburn, and you've allowed me to monopolise you when you should be back inside with your family. In fact, we both need to get back before they send out a search party!"

Alex assured her that he'd enjoyed chatting to her and learning about her work. He would willingly talk to her again, he told her, for all the time she could spare.

They walked back together, separating when Erin was pulled

away on some errand as soon as she was spotted by another member of staff. Alex headed back to Beth, Anna and Simon, and met Trish Gartner on her way out.

She smiled at him and he heard once again a low voice whispering, *'pat-a-cake,'* as he did every time he encountered her at the engineering works, sounding like a soft breeze rustling late autumn leaves. All this time he hadn't been sure whether it was male or female, but now he was certain it was a male voice, and that ruled out Trish's sister.

"Hello, Alex. I've been wondering if we'd ever bump into each other here. How's your wife's grandfather?" Trish asked.

"Oh, no change. How about your dad, how's he doing?"

"I can't believe he's still here. I don't want to sound callous, and I think you'll understand because of what you do, but I really wish he wouldn't hang on like this. He's almost a hundred and he's been bedbound and totally unaware of his surroundings for years. How on earth does the heart go on beating when the brain is so damaged with disease?"

"Do you believe in life after death, Trish?"

Trish gave a little laugh as she considered. "I think there are three kinds of people when it comes to that particular question, Alex. Those who, like you, believe one hundred per cent; those who say that death is the end of everything; and people like me who'd like to believe we continue in some form after we die yet can't quite get ourselves to do so."

Wanting to seize the opportunity to offer Trish some proof, Alex flexed his psychic senses, certain someone was trying to communicate with her through him. But the connection was still too weak and he could get nothing more so he had no choice but to leave it.

In bed that night, with Beth already fast asleep beside

him, Alex lay on his back, hands behind his head, wide awake because his mind was so busy running over and over what he'd witnessed at Rainstones House and the conversations he'd had that day with Kallie, Trish and Erin. Each one of them had given him a lot to think about.

Why had the couple with Kallie, who were most likely her grandparents, not tried to communicate with him? Why, too, did the person saying *'pat-a-cake'* when he was with Trish not answer him when he acknowledged that he could hear him? And then there was Erin's question going round and round in his head about some of her patients, the ones like Trish's father, Kallie's mother, and Simon: *where do they go?*

Chapter 25

By five o'clock Kallie had tidied up the treatment room so it was clean and ready to use by the next day's therapists. She changed out of her matching tunic and trousers into shirt and jeans then, grabbing her bag and jacket, raced to the canteen for coffee and a chat with Trish before they both went to the dementia wing.

Trish was already seated at a table by the window, two large slices of cake in front of her.

"I got chocolate and this one is coconut. Do you have a particular preference or shall we have half of each?"

"Half of each sounds good. I'll get the drinks, what'll you have?"

When they were settled they chatted about the guests they'd seen that day.

Trish said, "The new guest turned out to be a real live wire and comedian who had everyone in stitches. It's the joyful and positive days like today that keep me coming back week after week. How about you, you had a busy day, didn't you?"

"Yes, I did, practically back to back appointments. My nose is so full of aromatherapy oils this coffee smells like perfume!" She took a sip and pulled a face. "Tastes like it, too!

I was thinking how sad it is that all those DPU guests I met on my first day eighteen months ago are gone. And with my mother in the dementia wing . . . well, life takes some strange turns, doesn't it?"

She took a mouthful of the coconut cake as Trish agreed with her that life was, indeed, strange, then said, "Trish, can I ask you something? That tall, good looking man, Alex, I was talking to him last week and he said he knows you. Are you good friends with him, by any chance?"

Trish laughed. "I hope you don't have designs on him, Kallie Harper, because he's very much married and it would break Kevin's heart to learn your affections lie elsewhere. We're not personal friends, I work for him."

Trish raised her eyebrows and Kallie explained, "Erin told me that he's a psychic medium on the telly, do you have something to do with that, then?"

"Oh no, not at all. Remember I told you I had a part time job in a steel engineering works? Well, Alex is the owner. I don't see him there often, though, he's too busy with the TV show and his books and stuff. That's why he doesn't come to visit his wife's grandfather all that often, either. I have to admit he scared me a little the first few times I met him, I always wondered if he was reading my mind or something, but he's a lovely guy and so friendly. So, come on, why are you asking me about him?"

Kallie expelled a breath and told Trish she wanted to tell her the whole story but it would take far too long if they were to get over and see their respective parents.

"Kallie, they don't even know we're there! It sounds as if this is important to you, so let's replenish our coffees and you tell me what's on your mind. You must consider me a friend or you wouldn't have told me all about your relationship with your mother and your grandparents. If it would help you to talk about whatever's bothering you now then I'm more than happy to listen."

Kallie took a deep breath and told Trish about the strange things that happened in her house. She had the electrics checked out and everything was fine. Things had settled down for a little while, but then, about the time she learned that Celia was coming to Rainstones House, it had started up again and lasted for a couple of weeks. She'd had quite a period of respite but now it was active one more and although it didn't scare her it did make her wonder as to the cause of it.

"After my grandparents died it was things like the television changing channels or suddenly the volume going really loud, lights going on and off, items going missing only to turn up again when I'd searched absolutely everywhere." She told Trish then about the time the perfume bottle had tipped off the dressing table and filled the room with her grandmother's scent. "I used to joke out loud, telling Walter and Verity to pack it in. When my mum came to stay that time she broke her wrist she said she heard voices and saw shadows. I haven't heard voices but I do see shadows sometimes.

"Well, as I say, since Mum's condition got worse the weird happenings have started up again, and I can't say exactly why I think this, but I'm really beginning to suspect that it might be my grandparents and they may be trying to tell me something. If it isn't them, I think I need some help to find out what's going on. I thought of approaching Alex if he was a friend of yours, but if he's somebody famous he's not likely to have time for me, is he?"

"Wow, Kallie, I certainly wasn't expecting all that. It actually sounds quite exciting, though I'm not sure I'd like to spend a night at your place! Your cottage is next to a graveyard, isn't it?"

She dabbed up the last of the chocolate cake crumbs from the plate and licked them from her finger as she considered Kallie's problem. "I'm on the fence when it comes to life after death and all that stuff, but do you really think it could be your grandparents? Alex is very approachable, you know. You've spoken to him, haven't you? Well then, you know he's not at all the arrogant celebrity type that plays on his fame, and I think you should talk to him. If he can't help you directly then maybe he can give you some advice. It's worth a try."

"I suppose. But I don't know that I can just go up and ask him."

Trish laughed and told her she'd just have to, or she'd regret the missed opportunity. She checked the time and said they could still go to the dementia unit for a few minutes.

Feeling bloated, Kallie regretted that she'd eaten so much cake and Trish laughed, saying she felt the same. The cakes in the canteen were really portioned far too generously, but they were irresistible.

When they got to the dementia unit, Trish went to her father's room and Kallie looked for Celia, but there was no sign of her. Sitting in the far corner, as if she'd conjured him up by wishing it, was Alex Kelburn. He was sitting with his wife and it looked like Simon Savarese was having a quiet episode, because Alex and Beth were just talking quietly between themselves. Unable to figure out how to approach him, Kallie decided to let it go for now and go on home.

Trish appeared at that moment. "Dad's fast asleep so there's no point in staying. I see Alex is over there, aren't you going to speak to him?"

"Oh, I can't, Trish! Look, he's with his wife. I can't just march up to him, can I?"

"Well, I don't know how else you're going to do it, unless you want me to ask him for you? Oh, he's seen us. Come on, Kallie, don't run away."

Kallie's elbow was held firmly by Trish as Alex approached them. Heavens, he was handsome, in that slightly dishevelled way that she liked.

"Hello Trish, Kallie. How are you both?"

They both replied at the same time, then Trish said that Kallie needed to ask him something. Horrified and embarrassed at being put on the spot Kallie glowered at her, but Alex gave a friendly smile as if waiting for her to speak, so she decided it was now or never. She managed to choke out that she was having a problem with her house and she thought it might be haunted.

"Is it frightening you, or do you think someone's just trying to get your attention?"

"Um, a bit of both? It's been happening on and off since my grandparents died. They both went within months of each other, my grandmother actually died in the cottage so . . . maybe it's them? I'm sorry to bother you with this, I'm sure you're far too busy." Cheeks flaming, she tried to back away to make her escape, but Trish tightened her grip on Kallie's arm.

"Not at all," said Alex. "I can see your grandparents with you, Kallie, and as we're speaking I'm getting a good idea of what's going on." He turned to Trish. "And someone is also trying to get through to you, too, Trish, but it's too weak for me to work out who it is yet."

"Really?" Kallie and Trish squeaked together.

Alex grinned. "I usually close down my psychic senses

when I'm out and about otherwise I get bombarded, but I'm certainly aware of loved ones being with both of you. It will be too difficult to have any kind of communication here and it would help me to come to your house, so would you like me to do that? Trish could come along too, if that's okay with both of you?"

Kallie stuttered that she couldn't possibly impose on Alex in that way, but upon his and Trish's insistence she finally gave him her address and they arranged a date and time for him to be there.

He went back to his wife and Simon, leaving Kallie and Trish looking open-mouthed at each other, astonished that they were going to get the personal services of a highly renowned psychic medium, whether or not they fully believed in what he did.

Chapter 26

"What's happening? Dad? Dad! Where are you going?"

Hearing Anna call out, Erin moved in sharply as Simon evaded Anna's grip, and called to another nurse to come and help.

"Take him out, Raina. Let me talk to Mrs Savarese."

Raina had to chase after Simon, as he was surprisingly fast on his feet but when she caught up with him, she gently steered him safely out of the room without touching him.

"Is this the first time you've seen him go walkabout?" Erin said to Anna. "Don't worry, Raina is taking him to the safe area where he can move unimpeded and without danger to himself." She placed her hand on Anna's trembling arm. "This happens, we don't know why. It's as if they are driven by some inner impulse and they simply must move. It's recognised these days that it helps to just let them move freely, as long as they are safe, and not try to restrain them."

Anna finally found her voice. "How long has he been doing this? How long will it last?"

"To answer your first question, it started a couple of days ago. I can't say how long it will last I'm afraid, because there's no time limit. Sometimes they walk for ten or twenty minutes, sometimes it's for hours. Sometimes they'll come back and sit quietly, other times they need to be put to bed because they are exhausted. It's distressing to see, I know, but your dad is safe, I promise you."

Erin could see that Anna was fighting back tears at how fast this appalling thing was happening to her father as she said, "He doesn't even know us anymore. Should I stay and wait to see if he comes back?"

"I would suggest you go home. If you like I can make sure someone calls you later so you know he's okay and resting, but I do assure you that he'll be fine. All of us are used to these situations, so your dad will be well taken care of no matter how long he feels compelled to walk."

"I hate this bloody disease so much," whispered Anna, her face crumpling.

"I know, believe me, I know how upsetting this is. I saw your daughter here earlier, has she gone? Is anyone else coming? In that case perhaps you should go and have a cup of tea before you leave, steady yourself before driving home."

Trish appeared then just behind Anna, having spent half an hour with her father. He was very ill now and Erin knew that Trish was desperate for it to be over. They all wanted it to be over, for the poor man and his family deserved the release his death would bring after all these years. At least, Erin thought, as far as they could tell he had never been in any pain.

"I'm sorry, but I couldn't help overhearing. I'm Trish. I'm about to go to the cafeteria before going home, would you like to come with me? I could do with the company."

Erin smiled at her, saying to Anna, "I think that's a great idea. I'll go and check on your father and ask someone to call you later to tell you how he is. Okay?"

Mutely, Anna nodded her head and went with Trish.

Erin, going to see if Simon was still merrily sundowning, thought to herself how, in all her years as a nurse, she must have witnessed just about every type of family dynamic. The Savareses were a very loving and close-knit family, supporting each other all the time. Trish too had close family, with a super husband and four strapping sons who teased her mercilessly and clearly loved her deeply, and all the members of her extended family who came when they could. Then there was young Kallie, coping all alone with a mother she hardly knew.

***

As if from a long way away, Simon was conscious of a babble of voices and of being touched by unseen hands, but it felt like he'd been anaesthetised and all his senses were numb. He wanted to speak, but he couldn't get his throat and tongue to form the words. Nothing made sense to him except the sudden, overwhelming urge to move, just to walk and walk and walk until exhaustion took him back into deep sleep and the beautiful dreams he treasured.

Oh, it felt so good to be on the move! To feel the oxygen filling his lungs and the blood pumping round his body, to feel his muscles flex, the tendons stretch and contract. He was vaguely aware that he was going round in circles in an empty room, the carpet and walls different shades of green, the ceiling summer blue, so it almost felt like he was outside.

He sensed, too, that he was not alone, that another paced with him, breathing hard, muttering things Simon couldn't make out, and there was someone standing by the door, arms crossed, like a sentinel. But he didn't want to see or hear anyone else. He didn't want anyone or anything to encroach on this glorious feeling of freedom, because he knew in his soul that if he could just go fast enough he'd go to where he really wanted to be.

Yes! The green beneath his feet changed from carpet to real, sweet grass. The walls and ceiling receded and he was walking beneath real blue skies, the colours so intense he wanted to laugh out loud at the sheer beauty of it. Now he could slow down, now he could stroll at leisure and smell the perfumes wafting in the air, hear the birdsong, feel the warmth of that strange purple-hued sun on his skin.

He'd been here many times before and knew where to go.

Eventually he saw the high wall in the distance, the length of it running side to side as far as the eye could see and beyond. When he'd come across it the first time he'd thought it was an impenetrable barrier, but then he had seen the gate. And behind the gate had been Sylvia, but it was padlocked and neither of them could get it open. He'd kept coming and at last the chain had fallen away and they had simply looked at each other in wonderment.

In the early times, something had always drawn him back before they had spoken a word and he'd felt each time that his heart would break to be torn from her so soon. Lately, the times they had together seemed longer and they would sit together and talk, yet it was never long enough and all too soon he was pulled back again.

There she was! She was seated on the grass as always, her back against the great stone wall, her face raised to the sun.

"Sylvia!" His voice echoed as he broke into a run, her name rebounding off the sun-warmed stones of the wall.

She looked up, her face breaking into a wide, joyful smile,

and she rose to meet him. She wore a necklace of small white flowers with pink centres, and seeing how fresh, how lovely she looked, Simon ran even faster.

Within moments he had closed the gap and clasped her outstretched hands. She looked so young and he felt so young. For eons, they stared at each other, communicating with hearts, minds and souls. Oh, how he loved this woman, his Sylvia, his true soulmate.

Without speaking and without letting go of hands, they sank down to the ground, cushioned by the warm, green grass. This is where he wanted to be, where he needed to be, and he knew Sylvia felt the same. She waited for him here, she'd told him, she would always wait for him. The barrier behind them would never keep them apart again, for she would not go back through the gate until the time came when he could pass through it with her.

He leaned forward until their lips met in a long, loving kiss. He told her how much he loved her and that he wouldn't leave her again.

"I made a daisy chain for you," she said, holding it out to him.

Laughing, he bowed his head to receive it, but before she could place it round his neck he felt it. The tug, that irresistible force pulling him back, dragging him away from Sylvia.

"No!"

Her expression changed to one of confusion and then alarm. She threw the daisies down and reached out for him but he was already too far away to touch her. He managed only to scream her name and to promise he would be back, and then, once more, his eyes were looking at carpet and walls and ceiling. The sentinel was still there in the doorway. Simon stumbled and pitched forward with an anguished cry.

Chapter 27

Leaning back in his chair, Alex was feeling rather pleased with himself as he flexed his fingers and stretched his spine. He'd risen early and spent a couple of productive hours editing his book and then he'd worked through the never-ending pile of letters that continued to flood in, more than doubling since the programme about Rachel and Flora had been broadcast.

He had been saddened and frustrated that Rachel had been arrested shortly after his interview with her, but it hadn't come as a surprise to anyone. What had been a surprise was the reaction when the programme about her and Flora had been shown on television, because viewers and the press had gone mad for the story. There were even people protesting on Rachel's behalf because they believed in Alex! It could never make any difference to Rachel, but how humbling it was for him to know that some people had total trust and belief in his abilities.

Alex needed a break before continuing with the letters for another hour or so until he had to leave for the promised visit to Kallie's house. He ambled into the kitchen and fixed himself a mug of coffee and a thick roast beef and mustard sandwich. With the mug in one hand, a plate in the other and the newspaper tucked under his arm, he wondered if it was warm enough to sit outside or should he stay indoors? Deciding to test the outside temperature he used his elbow to push the door handle down, but a sudden jolt in his psychic senses made him all but drop everything he carried.

Someone had called his name, and it came in so loud, he physically winced. Carefully putting his burdens down, he stood stock still, allowing his senses to fully open. He had come to know this particular playful energy but he'd thought his role in getting her ready to move on was complete.

"Hello Flora. You gave me quite a start there! Almost spilled my coffee."

His mind filled with her giggle. She was so different to the shy, reticent little girl he'd first encountered at the edge of the shallow grave where her remains had lain buried.

"Are you all right, Flora? I wasn't expecting to keep hearing from you now you've settled things with your mum."

"I miss her."

"I know you do. She misses you, too."

Alex waited for the little girl to ask him how Rachel was coping with prison or to tell him why she was coming through, but she said nothing.

"Is there something else you want to tell me, Flora?"

"There's a lady with me. She wants to talk to you."

"Oh? Is she related to you? Can you tell me her name?"

Alex had always hoped that Flora wasn't alone, that she was with some family members; maybe this was one of them with something to say to him. The silence continued for so long that Alex began to wonder if Flora had broken the connection. Then...

"Alex? Alex, can you hear me? It's Sylvia"

Sylvia. At last!

Beth asked him constantly why he hadn't been able to make contact with her and he'd tried and tried, but until this moment he'd not even caught the merest scent of her.

There was that time after the fire, when Simon had whispered to him that he'd seen her, that he had expected her to make contact with him, but she hadn't. Simon had subsequently told him a couple of times more that he went to the place Sylvia was, and Alex had kept that to himself until he could be sure of what was happening. If Simon had said that Sylvia visited him, Alex would have understood it, but Simon was certain that he went to Sylvia, not the other way round.

This left Alex trying to figure out how Simon could go to the Other Side when he was still very much alive, and it made him think again of Erin's question. At no point had Simon come even close to dying in that fire, so it made no sense. And how come Sylvia was with Flora?

"It's so good to hear from you, Sylvia. I have no idea how you and Flora found each other, but I'm so glad you have."

"Grace brought her to me. She was alone here, waiting to see her mother, or get a message to her. I thought she would leave me once that was done, but she seems to want to stay and now she's helped me to make a link with you."

"Are you alright, Sylvia? Is Grace still with you?"

"Oh yes, I'm fine, but I've rarely seen Grace since she brought Flora to me. I never dreamed the likes of Grace existed, but there are many like her here. Are they angels? She told me about your accident, in fact she showed me what you and your friend Scott saw, the kingfisher catching a golden fish, remember? I watched it just as you did Alex, all in that wonderful slow motion so you could see every detail. I saw it all and it was so beautiful."

Oh yes, Alex remembered. How could he forget? He had

included it in the book he was currently writing, how he'd seen the beautiful, iridescent kingfisher plunging like a dart, creating a crown of water that rose up, sparkling in the sunlight, before separating into silvery beads that fell gently back down again. The bird had reappeared, glittering droplets cascading, with a small golden fish wriggling in its beak. A hundred shimmering rainbows had hovered in the air until his friend Scott had sighed with the acceptance of his death, knowing in that moment that he would continue to exist.

He asked Sylvia how she was adjusting to her new existence. She laughed.

"Only you could ask me that! It's different than anything I'd ever dreamed. In fact, I'm not sure I ever dreamed anything about what came after dying. It's . . . oh! It's like trying to describe a rainbow to someone who's never seen colour, isn't it?"

"Yes, I know just what you mean. Sylvia, these links can be hard to maintain when you're new to it, so what can I do for you? Do you know what's going on with Simon? Am I to tell Anna, Beth and Paul that we've talked?"

Sylvia told him that the only thing she knew was that she needed to remain where she was to be there whenever Simon came. Though his visits were brief, they meant everything to her.

This so startled Alex that he found himself gripping the table's edge. Sylvia was confirming what Simon had said. But what did she mean by whenever Simon came?

"Simon told me he visits you. I don't understand."

"You've been here, Alex, isn't it the same thing?"

"I'm not sure that it is. I was badly injured in that accident, pretty close to dying in fact, but Simon was merely a little burnt in the fire. He's very much alive Sylvia, so I can't see how he comes over to where you are."

"But he does come, just not for very long. He sits with me and we talk for a while, then he seems to be pulled away against his will. He doesn't want to go, he wants to stay with me in this wonderful place where we're both young again and so happy. Why can't he stay Alex, do you know?"

His mind raced. If Sylvia did not visit her family then perhaps she didn't know that Simon was in a dementia care home. Should he tell her? He was still trying to formulate a reply when it dawned on him that the link had been broken, and he could only surmise that Sylvia had depleted her energy. Tutting with frustration, Alex reached out to Flora, but she had gone too.

Abandoning his coffee, which was now cold anyway, he decided to see if he could contact his father. He opened his mind again and called, but instead of the warm and gentle male energy he expected he was blasted with such force he exclaimed out loud and had to hold his head in his hands until the energy lessened enough to allow him to think.

"Have you understood yet, Alex?" the familiar female voice said.

Not knowing what she meant but knowing full well that she would offer no explanation, Alex replied that he didn't know what it was he was meant to understand. He waited, watching Grace take form in the room like a static tornado until he could see her tall figure and startling black eyes in front of him.

"It's all laid out for you Alex, you just need to work it out. You know that those who have crossed over can communicate with their loved ones for you are a bridge between the two worlds, but now you are asking yourself why it is that Sylvia can be visited by her husband when he is still very much alive. There are others around you that are able to do the same thing. Who is it that calls 'pat-a-cake'? Why are Kallie's grandparents trying to get her attention, is

it something to do with Kallie's mother, their daughter? Think it through, Alex. It is important that you understand, for you must explain to others."

And she was gone, with Alex muttering that things would be far simpler if should would just tell him what she wanted him to know and not talk in riddles.

Feeling winded and confused with what had just happened, Alex glanced at his watch and realised he ought to get going if he was going to make it to Kallie's at the agreed time.

* * *

Kallie waited with Trish, feeling ridiculously nervous. "Maybe he's not going to come?"

"He's only ten minutes late, Kallie. Did you catch his programme the other night about the little girl whose remains were found on a building site?" When Kallie shook her head she continued, "It was amazing, truly amazing. I see him in a whole new light now; you must see it if you can."

They both heard a car draw up, then a door slamming, followed by footsteps coming up the path. There was a sharp rap on the door.

"See?" said Trish. "Now calm down and let him in."

Alex had to duck slightly as he came through the low door, apologising for being late. Kallie dismissed his apologies, saying she was grateful that he'd agreed to come at all. She went to make coffee, listening from the kitchen as Trish talked to him about the latest goings-on at his factory. It seemed an odd combination, Kallie thought, an engineering works and TV psychic medium, but then again, what kind of job would go alongside being a psychic medium?

She carried the drinks through and sat next to Trish, not having a clue what would come next. She'd meant to see if she could get one of his TV shows on her laptop but had put it off and put if off until it was too late, and she hadn't known about the programme Trish had just mentioned. Now here he was, Alex Kelburn, in her living room, about to give her and Trish a personal reading.

"Trish, I said someone is trying to make contact with you. Unfortunately, it's a really weak connection. At first, I thought it might be your sister, but now I'm pretty sure it's a man. What I hear is 'pat-a-cake' does that mean anything to you?"

Trish gave an incredulous laugh. "It was what my dad called me! Everyone else calls me Trish, but to Dad I was always his 'pat-a-cake'. I was his youngest, you see, and I think he spent more time with me as I was growing up than he did with any of my half siblings."

Alex frowned. "I'm confused by this, Trish, but I think it is your dad that I hear. I just don't understand how, though. He is still alive, isn't he?"

Trish nodded. "Yes, but he's not at all well. He's definitely fading and we're taking it day by day."

"Hmm. But I first heard it when you started working at the factory and no matter how hard I've tried I just can't get anything else. Let me work with Kallie now and we'll see if anything else comes up for you. Kallie, on my way over here I was getting that you've had the television and lights going on and off and strange phone calls. Tell me what's been happening here that led you to want to talk to me about it."

Still feeling nervous, and wondering just how Alex knew about the strange goings-on and how much he was going to charge for this meeting, Kallie went through the timeline of events. As she explained about the electrics misbehaving and items going missing and reappearing, and the time her grandmother's perfume bottle fell to the floor, suddenly it all sounded so ridiculous, so trivial. But Alex was listening intently, his focus entirely on her. Eventually her tale was told, and she tailed off not knowing what else to say.

After a silence she realised that Alex was no longer looking at her, but at a point just over her right shoulder.

"Verity," he said. "And Walter. They're here, Kallie."

Trish muttered, "Bloody hell," and when Kallie glanced at her she wasn't sure if her friend was excited, amused or scared.

"As you've told me so much, Kallie, I'm asking for something evidential that they can tell me, something I couldn't know. The most trivial details are usually the ones that provide the most compelling evidence. Ah! You didn't mention the mysterious phone calls? Your gran is telling me that they found they were able to make the phone ring but realised they couldn't speak through it and it was annoying you. Walter is telling me that before he died he sent you out to make a pot of tea. He hopes you weren't too upset, but he really wanted to be alone with Verity when he took his last breath. It's a promise they'd made to each other. Verity says she told you that Walter was always with her in the months leading up to her own death, and he really was. They'd both known that Verity was ill but they had decided not to tell you."

Kallie swallowed back the tears that threatened. Was it really possible that her grandparents were talking to Alex, as if they were in the room?

After a short pause Alex spoke again. "Your grandparents raised you. You and your mother have never been able to get on, but they say you were wrong about her and they wish you could have seen that. Um, wait, Verity is showing me something."

Alex closed his eyes and Kallie could only stare stupidly at him while she waited for whatever was coming next.

"She's showing me a box of wine glasses." He hesitated, eyes still closed. "You have to wash them. You're angry with your mother because she hasn't been helping you, and when she says something about the glasses. It escalates into an argument." He opened his eyes. "Verity was watching you both and it made her very sad because your mother left so quickly after that."

He went on and on, telling her snippets of things that had happened in a way that left her in no doubt that Verity and Walter were giving him the information. She was crying openly now, and so was Trish, who rummaged in her bag for tissues for both of them to mop their tears and blow their noses.

"They were watching over Celia too, and knew about her diagnosis and what she was planning. But there's something I'm missing," said Alex finally. "Not for you, but for me. I'm supposed to understand something from all this, so I need to go away and think about it. All I can tell you at this stage, Kallie, Trish, is that your loved ones are around you and they have a specific and important message that is as much for me as it is for you that I can't quite get hold of. If you don't mind, I'll leave you now and I'll be in touch when I've worked it all out."

He beamed at both women and Trish thought she might melt at his handsomeness. What a lovely, lovely man!

When she found her voice to offer him another drink, which he declined, she then blushed furiously as she asked him what she owed him.

"Owe me?" He blinked in incomprehension, then laughed, throwing his head back. "Oh, I see! Your grandparents are highly amused at your discomfort, Kallie. I don't want any money from either of you, it's been my pleasure. I think, I know that all this is for my benefit too, though just what that benefit might be is currently hidden from me. I bid you good day, ladies, and if I don't see you at Rainstones House, I'll call you."

When he'd gone, Kallie made more coffee for her and Trish and they talked about how amazing and gorgeous Alex was and dissected what they both thought was one of the most fascinating couple of hours they'd ever spent.

"What do you make of it, Kallie? He seemed to be giving you a lot of information that he couldn't have known."

Kallie nodded. "I know. It was astonishing! I had hoped it was Gran and Grandad and now I know it is I feel just great." She looked all around the room and spoke up to the ceiling, "Thank you Verity and Walter! Feel free to visit any time, I love you both so much!"

Trish laughed. "He didn't have much for me, though."

Kallie asked about the 'pat-a-cake' and Trish explained again how it had been her father's nickname for her for as long as she could remember.

"But he's not dead, so it can't be him. I was wondering if it's my grandfather, though I never knew him. I wonder what Alex meant when he said there was an important message in all this for him too? Imagine being able to communicate with the dead. What must that be like?"

"I'd quite like it I think," said Kallie. "At least, I'd like to be able to see and talk to my grandparents again."

Chapter 28

The familiar scrawled writing had Kallie taking the proffered envelope with some trepidation.

"Where did this come from, Erin? It's my mother's writing so she must have done this ages ago."

"It was given to Sasha for safekeeping when Celia arrived here and she handed it to me yesterday to pass on to you when you came in. There was another letter with it explaining how she wanted things to be handled and why. I hope you don't mind but I have seen that accompanying letter as it was addressed to the staff of the dementia unit who had direct dealings with your mother, and Sasha particularly thought it might help me to read it before I gave this sealed envelope to you. Apparently, your mother knew just what might happen and wanted you to have it if, or when, she became unable to recognise you."

She gave a gentle smile and patted Kallie's hand. "I'm sorry that happened so quickly after she arrived, Kallie. There's no knowing how fast dementia will progress, and exactly which of the many symptoms each person will experience."

"Maybe it's just as well she's no longer aware because now she doesn't know what's happening to her, does she?"

"There's no way of knowing, Kallie. From what I've learned your mum had it all worked out from the moment she even suspected something was wrong. She didn't know if you would visit her, and she said she would understand if you didn't and no one was to judge you for it. From what you've told me you two certainly had a difficult relationship."

Kallie sighed. "That we did."

She smoothed the fabric of her tunic with one hand, looking down at the thick envelope she held in her other hand. After a long pause, she switched her gaze back to Erin, who was regarding her fondly and with so much sympathy Kallie was in danger of bursting into tears.

"Do you know what's in it?"

Erin shook her head and told her the envelope had remained sealed by the solicitor's stamp as it was meant for Kallie's eyes only.

"I know it was awkward when she arrived and you found visiting her such a strain, but you kept coming and I'm sure in my heart that she appreciated it. As I say, no-one but Celia knows what's in that envelope and as she's given every other detail a great deal of thought then I imagine this is important. I suggest you take it home, take the phone off the hook, maybe pour yourself a glass of wine, and open it when you are ready. Maybe it will help you understand her a little, Kallie, or maybe it's nothing more than her funeral instructions." She placed her hand over Kallie's and gave it a light squeeze. "There's only one way to find out."

Kallie gave a short, mirthless laugh. "God. I can hardly take it in. All my life my mother has surprised me, and not usually in a good way, and now this. I hardly knew her really, and seeing her struggle with dementia has just about broken my heart, because the chance for us to make peace with each other has well and truly gone. Maybe—probably—neither of us would have taken that chance anyway, who knows? But it's so desperately sad to see such a brilliant mind wiped out. In a strange way, I do miss her."

"Of course you miss her. Parents and children may not always see eye to eye, I've had a few fall outs with my own kids, but the bond is always there. Just you keep on coming and sitting with her, because I do believe that at some level she knows you are there. Now then, I need to get home. It's been a long day and I need my cup of tea the way only my husband can make it. I hope whatever's in that envelope brings you some sense of peace. I'll see you soon, okay?"

Kallie smiled, loving this thoughtful, kind and generous nurse, and glad that it had been Erin entrusted to pass on the letter. The other nurses were truly wonderful, but Erin was extra special in Kallie's eyes, and she knew Trish felt the same. She would do as Erin suggested, go home, lock the doors, have some wine, switch off her phone, and open this last communication she was ever likely to get from her mother.

***

The envelope had been sealed with a thick circle of red wax and Kallie struggled to prise the flap open and keep the envelope intact. Celia had scrawled across the front: Strictly Private & Confidential. Only to be opened by Kathleen Harper.

Kathleen. That hated name. But did she hate it really? Hadn't she changed it to even further distance herself from her mother? She'd always blamed Celia for the deep flaws in their relationship, but now, too late, she was beginning to realise that once she'd reached adulthood and been able to reason things out, she had to take her share of the blame for the sometimes-awful way they'd behaved in each other's company.

She heaved a sigh, trying to picture Celia writing this shortly after she'd received the dreadful diagnosis. She could imagine the scientist in her taking over, that deep need to research, to analyse, to know as much as there was to know.

How sad, though, how dreadful, that she had learned of it just weeks after she'd returned to Cambridge once her broken arm had sufficiently healed so she could look after herself. She had never told Kallie, keeping her in the dark until just days before she'd moved into Rainstones House.

To say she had been stunned and confused at her mother's arrival in the dementia care wing was an understatement, but her mother had arrived and Kallie had gone to see her that evening. Celia had been okay then, you'd hardly know she had anything wrong with her apart from some absent-mindedness and the constant hand-wringing that Kallie had never seen before, but the respite had been short and with the benefit of hindsight, Kallie had realised too late that her mother's strange and erratic behaviour while she was staying at the cottage with her was due to the onset of the disease.

The flap came open at last, with just a little tear at the edge where the wax seal was so firmly stuck. She extracted several thick sheets of writing paper, pale cream like the envelope, each page covered both sides in her mother's tight, untidy handwriting. Kallie reached for her glass of wine and settled back to read.

***

After a night of tossing and turning, Kallie gave up trying

to sleep as soon as the dawn chorus started. Rising from her bed, she said good morning to Walter and Verity, wishing with all her heart that she could see them like Alex Kelburn did because it felt as if she'd never needed them as much as she did now. Alex's visit had clarified many things for her, but had her grandparents known about the letter? Well, if they hadn't, perhaps they'd both been reading it over her shoulder last night.

Had they cried as much as she had? God, she'd hardly been able to read some of the lines. All her life she'd seen her mother as this remote figure who hadn't wanted her and would have palmed her off to strangers if Verity and Walter hadn't intervened. She'd thought her unfeeling and unloving, argumentative and difficult. She'd hated her for not telling her who her father was. Well, she'd never know now who he was now and it didn't matter. It really didn't.

Kallie had enjoyed a wonderful childhood, but instead of recognising that it was thanks to her mother, who had made sure of it by allowing her to be raised by two people who knew how to be the kind of parents Kallie needed, the two people who had always understood her, she had seen it as a desertion of maternal duty. Celia had known her limitations, had known that she would not have made a good mother; it was simply the way she'd been made. But she had wanted the best for her daughter and had made sure she got it.

Never, not once, had Kallie thought of Celia as a person with a history that had little or nothing to do with her. Never had she considered how her mother thought, how she felt. Everything was coloured by the fractious relationship they'd had, and Kallie had laid the blame for that squarely on the shoulders of her mother.

What kind of a daughter had she been not to see beyond the

woman who cared nothing for appearances, the woman with a brilliant scientific mind who was revered in her field? Why had she never signed even a birthday or Christmas card for her?

Her mouth was so dry she could hardly swallow so she drank a large glass of fresh, cold water while the kettle boiled for tea. Trying to decide whether to go back to bed and drink the tea there, Kallie was instead drawn back to the couch, where the pages of Celia's letter still lay. How was she going to get through a day at the salon knowing what she now knew?

All this time she'd been visiting Celia it had been nothing more than a duty and now she was desperate to see her, just desperate to talk to her. Okay, Celia might not hear her and would not be able to respond in any case, but Kallie needed to talk to her. She needed to tell her mother how grateful she was, how sorry she was, how desperate she was that Celia should know that she loved her.

Chapter 29

For days Alex had been wrestling with his inability to decipher the messages contained in the readings he had given to Kallie and Trish. Or rather to Kallie, because he'd been unable to tell Trish anything much.

Kallie's grandmother had told him something that she didn't want Kallie to know yet, that Celia was sometimes with them, watching over Kallie in the cottage or when she was working or visiting in Rainstones House. He'd asked Verity how that could be when Celia was alive but they hadn't had an answer to that.

"She's here with us sometimes. That's all I can tell you, Alex. But she doesn't think Kallie should know this, at least not yet. Celia wrote a letter for her when she first got the diagnosis and she wants to see what Kallie's reaction is to that."

Baffled, Alex had kept this gem to himself when he'd been talking to Kallie and Trish in Kallie's living room, but he couldn't help comparing this to Sylvia telling him that Simon was sometimes with her. What was happening? How could it be happening? Had Kallie received her mother's letter yet, and what did it contain?

A glance at the alarm clock showed him it was ten past three in the morning and though he had a busy day ahead of him he knew he just had to get up and think about it all while Beth was sleeping, before the working day began and he would have no time to himself.

Rising quietly so as not to disturb Beth, he fumbled his way downstairs in the dark until he reached his study. Snapping on the light he sat at his desk, took a ruler and a sharp pencil from the drawer and pulled a pad of paper towards him.

"Okay," he muttered. "Let's work this out."

He started by writing 'Rainstones House' at the top of the page, then he divided the page into three columns. In the left column, he listed the names of those on the Other Side he'd had recent communication with, leaving a large gap between each name: Verity and Walter, the 'pat-a-cake' man, Sylvia, Flora. In the middle column, he wrote the names of the Rainstones residents who connected with the names in the first column: Celia Harper, Trish's father, Simon.

In his third column, he wrote the names of the living who were most closely connected with the other two columns: Kallie Harper, Trish, Anna. Frowning at Flora because her connection was purely to Sylvia and had nothing to do with anyone in Rainstones he decided he could cross out her name as she didn't figure in this conundrum.

He joined the families with more lines, arrows and circles while his brain absorbed what he was seeing written on the paper. The message he needed to know was in there, he knew it as sure as he knew his own name, but what was he missing?

"You're up early, Alex."

"Dad! Have you come to help me?"

There was a warm chuckle.

"I've struggled alongside you to work this out, but now I've had inside information and know the missing piece."

Alex sat up with a start. "What? You know what this all means? Then for heaven's sake tell me!"

"I'm not the one who solved the puzzle. Alistair did, and he's here to tell you."

Laughing, Alex threw down his pen and rubbed his tired eyes.

"Hello Uncle Alistair. Did you find your lady?"

Alistair confirmed that he had indeed found her, his gorgeous Jeanie. They had enjoyed an ecstatic reunion and Jeanie had told him that she'd always thought he would have moved on and found another, but she'd felt his presence and his undiminished love for her the minute he'd set out to look for her and had come a long way back to be with him.

"She said it was like a slight vibration at first, and then a compulsion to go to this place she'd never seen before and hadn't been aware of. We met by a gate Alex, an ornate, wrought iron gate set into a high stone wall that seemed to go on forever. At first, I could see only her, my Jeanie, but she said there were others there waiting, lots of others. After a while I could see them, but it was like looking through layers of film, each layer containing all these people, but they were unaware of each other in the different layers. I wondered if Sylvia might be there, in one of those layers, so I set my thoughts to finding her and I did!"

This made goosebumps break out all over Alex's body and he gave an involuntary shiver. This news was amazing, fantastic, wonderful!

Alistair talked some more, describing the scene by the mysterious gate while Alex stared at his piece of paper. He said Simon had appeared while he was with Sylvia and he'd left them to their reunion.

"It was short, though. I went back to Jeanie and when I turned around Sylvia was alone. She said it didn't matter, she knew Simon would be back. As long as she waited by that gate, she told me, he would always know where to find her and one day he would be able to stay for good. On that day, they would pass through the gate together."

And then Alex got it, the realisation slamming into him like a sledgehammer smashing through concrete. The pencil in his hands snapped in two and he couldn't stop himself from yelling out with joy, which woke up Beth who came running down, her hair wild, her eyes wide, asking what the hell was wrong?

"I'm sorry I woke you, but Beth, my goodness, I can see it now! I can see what's been going on with Simon!"

Blinking the sleep from her eyes Beth pulled out the other office chair and sat down. She pulled her dressing gown tightly around her and said, "Tell me."

Pointing to his columns on the page he talked her through it. "Look here, it's a bit of a mess now with all my doodles, but see where I've drawn the lines? Sylvia said that Simon visits her but can't stay. Kallie's grandparents said that Celia Harper is sometimes with them, and they are all watching over Kallie, but then she goes away again. Trish's father, the only one who's ever called her 'pat-a-cake' communicates that one word to me every time I'm near her, yet he is in a near-coma at Rainstones."

Beth scratched her head. "Okay, I'm listening. Keep going."

Alex leaned forward and took both her hands in his. "This is momentous, Beth."

The emotion that welled up in him came as a surprise, and he laughed as he wiped away some tears.

"Beth, people like Simon, like Celia Harper and Trish's dad, they are over there! They're on the Other Side! Do you see?

They are still living, but their spirit is somehow able to detach and pass over to where they can be with their loved ones! It makes sense, now I see it all. It's kind of what happens when we die: our spirit leaves the body and crosses over. In the case of dementia, and probably in cases of coma too, when they're as far gone as Simon and the others, the spirit detaches but it can't fully cross over and stay there permanently while the body still lives."

His face was alight. "Beth, Simon goes to Sylvia! I know this because she told me. When we see him sitting in that chair practically lifeless what we are seeing is just his body because he's not there—he's with Sylvia! They are together on the Other Side where they can touch each other and talk to other. Sylvia will wait there for him for as long as it takes for his time here to end, and then they will cross over together. And that's another thing I know. Their time here must be played out according to some unknown universal rule, it's just that in the meantime they are granted this special time in this wonderful waiting place on the Other Side."

Beth was laughing and crying now with joy at knowing Sylvia and Simon were sometimes together and Alex laughed too, thinking how wonderful, how magnificent it was, to know that Simon and the other dementia patients like him weren't trapped at all, they were free! Even if only for short periods of time, they were free, and they were happy.

Beth went to make them both some hot chocolate, leaving Alex staring at the piece of paper. He was about to follow her when he sensed a familiar, very powerful presence. He welcomed Grace, but she didn't speak, merely bowed her graceful head to him and he knew she was pleased with him. Alex bowed to her in return as she faded from sight, then another, weaker presence made itself felt and he had to flex his psychic muscles to make the connection. His smile grew wide as he realised who it was and why he had come.

***

Erin walked into the lounge to make sure everything was set for the quartet of female singers that were coming in after lunch to entertain the residents with songs from the 1930s and 1940s. It had been quite a day so far. Trish's father had died in the very early hours of the morning and Trish and her family had come straight away to say their goodbyes before his body had been taken away to the funeral home. Trish had cried a lot in the comfort of her husband's arms, but they had been tears of relief more than grief, and Erin knew she'd be fine.

Kallie had unexpectedly arrived at breakfast time too, seeking out Erin to tell her she'd read Celia's letter and wanted to talk to her mother in private. Suspecting that what was in that letter had been momentous for Kallie, Erin had taken her to Celia's room. She'd turned to leave but Kallie had asked to stay a moment.

"I know you're busy and you've got lots to do, I just wondered ..."

Erin had glanced at the cream envelope Kallie held out to her, recognising the handwriting on the front.

"Would you read it, Erin? Please? You look after her and apart from the very brief details she chose to share with anyone when she was diagnosed, you've no idea who she really was, just as I didn't. I honestly think she'd like you to read it, to know some important things about her life. And it would help me too to have another person, someone I trust, to share this with. If I'm asking too much, Erin, I'm sorry . . ." Kallie trailed off, embarrassed.

But Erin had been honoured and deeply moved at such a request, such trust. She had taken the letter and folded Kallie in her arms, promising that she would read it as soon as she could and return it. She let Kallie go, giving her a little shake as she looked deep into her eyes.

"Go and talk to Celia, Kallie. Talk to your mum and tell her how you feel."

Erin had left the room then, depositing the letter in her locker where it would be safe from prying eyes until she had the time to read it.

Now, having satisfied herself that all was ready for the band, Erin greeted the relatives and friends arriving to join their relatives for the entertainment.

Anna and Beth were among the last to arrive. The two women looking much brighter and more cheerful than Erin had ever seen them, took their usual places on either side of Simon. When they'd learned of the singalong, Anna had told Erin that Simon had an incredible memory for music and lyrics and she hoped that this would spark something in him.

He was always quiet these days, with the sundowning happening every day at the same time for the same length of time. Afterwards, he would go docilely to bed and sleep a straight ten hours.

Alex arrived and came straight over with a smile that made her heart flutter just a little. He really was good looking, and so endearing.

He said, "Erin, I know you're busy, but if you could spare me just a little time I'd like to talk to you. It's really important, so can we go and sit on the bench by the sculpture?"

Taken aback and wondering what on earth Alex Kelburn wanted to say to her that couldn't wait, Erin agreed. Asking another nurse to look after things in her absence, Erin grabbed her cardigan and followed Alex to the bench, stopping for a moment to smell the newly-mown grass. There had been a light shower in the early hours of the morning and everything felt so wonderfully fresh.

Alex asked her how she was.

"I'm fine and bursting with curiosity. But before you tell me why you want to speak to me; did you know Trish's father died this morning?"

He nodded. "He came and told me himself, Erin. He had a message for Trish which I will pass on to her as soon as I see her, but he also asked me to pass on a message to you."

Startled, Erin said doubtfully, "For me? Trish's dad?"

Alex gave her the message word for word and for a full minute Erin could only sit there, staring at him. Then she blinked and shook her head in wonder and said, "Is that why you asked to see me?"

"Not entirely, though that was part of it, of course. Do you remember the question you asked me when we sat here the first time?"

"Of course I do! We were talking about the patients who were no longer communicative in any way and I said I'd always wondered where they go."

Alex beamed at her, his dark eyes gleaming. "Well, that's what I really want to talk to you about." He took her hand and squeezed it. "Erin, I think you're going to love what I'm about to tell you."

After he'd finished imparting what he'd learned from Trish's father, Sylvia and his own Uncle Alistair, Erin was silent again for a long while, digesting it all. Then her face slowly lit up with delight and she leaned in to kiss Alex on the cheek.

"You are an amazing man, Alex Kelburn, and thank you is hardly enough for what you have just given me."

* * *

When Erin returned to the residents' lounge, she stood in the doorway for a moment taking in the scene that was so familiar yet now so different in the light of her new insight. To the sounds of wartime songs sung by the young women dressed up in smart military uniforms, her eyes roamed from armchair to armchair, alighting on all the patients she had come to care for so much. At one end of the spectrum were those who were like children, not knowing the year, the day or even the hour, but living cheerfully in the moment. At the other end were people like Celia and Simon, mostly present in body only, and it was these she could think of differently from now on, for she knew where their minds, their souls, actually were. And she knew that they were happy in that place and that they would remain there until their physical selves reached a natural end.

Yes, she wished there was no such disease as dementia, but as it did exist in its many and various forms and so many were afflicted, she could at least take comfort in all that Alex had explained to her out in the garden.

She couldn't help the slow, joyous smile as she recalled the message from Trish's father, who had wanted her to know that although his spirit had been quite far away for a very long time, he had always been aware of how well he'd been cared for. As if that wasn't wonderful enough, he had wanted to thank Erin most especially as she had treated him with care and devotion far above and beyond her duty.

How amazing, she thought to herself as she hurried forward to retrieve a precious lace handkerchief that had fallen from a lap, there is a place in the Afterlife reserved for all of her patients. A special place Alex had called 'The Waiting Gate' where they and others like them existed in happiness and contentment until their physical hearts stopped beating and they were ready to cross over completely.

The band started to sing *We'll Meet Again* inspiring many of the residents to sit up straighter and join in with smiles and shining eyes. How appropriate, thought Erin, as she took a chair and let her feet tap along with the music.

Part Five

THE LETTER

Chapter 30

My dear Kathleen,

As I sit here with pen and paper and write these opening words, I wonder if I will be able to say all I need to say, and if I'll then have the courage to let you see it. I wonder, too, how you will receive this, my first and last communication with you. Will you even read it, or will the sight of my handwriting on the envelope make you want to tear it up or toss it onto the fire unopened? We never could understand each other, so I can only hope and pray that you will give me this one last opportunity to explain myself. Please give yourself one last chance to get to know me as a person, and not just the mother you found so inadequate.

Learning I had vascular dementia came as a great shock, as I'm sure you can imagine, but I made sure to acquaint myself with the ins and outs of the illness so I could make preparations accordingly. I am not afraid, just sad at this particular exit from life.

I have a lot to say, a lot to explain, so to use a popular phrase, I hope you're sitting comfortably.

You may already know what I am going to tell you about

your grandparents and maternal great-grandparents, but do please indulge me as I give you a bit of history.

Your great-grandparents were of a generation who left the upbringing of their children to nannies, governesses and boarding schools. The boys were sent away at age seven and the girls were kept home to be taught piano, watercolour painting, embroidery and how to serve tea, having their domestic skills and quietude honed in order to attract a suitable husband. Mum told me she loved her childhood, for she loved her nanny, but when she fell in love with Walter he was considered beneath her because he was not of the landed gentry. They met when he was hired to repaint the nursery and attic rooms of the grand old house.

Mum was sixteen and she says it was love at first sight for both of them and they stole as many moments together as they could. He proposed and she told her parents one evening over dinner that she wanted to become engaged. It was not well received. Marry him, she was told, and you will be disinherited.

Mum made the only act of defiance I think she ever made, taking a few possessions and creeping out of the house in the early hours of a spring morning to elope. Time proved her right in her choice, did it not? A greater love match than Walter and Verity I have never seen, and I'm sure you feel the same way.

Mum hoped for a large family, envisaging lots of little Walters and Veritys that she would raise herself, but it was not to be, for not only was I to be their only child, it soon became very clear that I was not to be shaped in my mother's image at all, neither physically nor emotionally.

As I grew up, I had not the least interest in fashion and make-up, nor did I want to learn how to keep house, prepare meals and bake cakes, be always calm and demure like the perfect domestic Goddess that my mother was happy to be. No, I came into the world kicking and screaming, wanting to forge my own, very different path.

When I was young, Mum tried to interest me in being her little kitchen assistant, but I preferred to sit by myself and read books, which I could do, so I'm told, before anyone taught me. I'm sure this isn't true, but there's no doubt I was naturally gifted academically, and all I wanted was to fill my brain with learning. Domesticity was anathema to me; acquisition of knowledge an absolute joy and my life's purpose.

I cared nothing at all for outward appearances, and inevitably, while Mum was having her hair styled and set every Friday afternoon at the village hairdressers, I would walk there straight from school, sit on a chair and bury my nose in a text book. All subjects fascinated me, and I found them all so easy, especially maths, chemistry and physics.

In school sports I was a disaster, but it was more because I didn't want to play hockey or netball rather than I couldn't, so I was always the last to be picked for a team. But in anything scholastic I excelled, top of the class every time, and I know this made my parents both proud and bewildered. I tell you this not to boast, I am simply trying to paint you a picture of who I am.

I sailed through school easily and alone, having no need of friendships, and there was never any doubt that I was destined for university. Fortunately, Mum and Dad had recognised this possibility early on and started a savings account for my college fund, putting a little by every week. Mum made our clothes and made her housekeeping stretch every week, but she wanted to get a part-time job so they could put more money in the pot. Dad would not hear of it. He insisted that her place was in the home and his was being the sole breadwinner of the family, and that was that. They helped me achieve my ambition as much as they were able, and for this I am eternally grateful.

The years passed and I remained happily single as I studied for my degrees and my doctorate, then it came as no surprise to anyone when I announced that I would be devoting my life to the world of academia.

Mum and Dad resigned themselves to not being blessed with the grandchildren they so longed for. I genuinely had no interest in personal relationships and I made no effort to nurture friendships at school because I didn't feel the need.

Nor, when I reached adulthood, did I wish to be anyone's girlfriend. Dating meant having to make the effort to be attractive, about having to please another person, and I had seen the angst and torment amongst my teenaged peers at school as they worried themselves into extreme silliness over whether so-and-so liked them or not. Fortunately, it isn't the same now, but back then to be 'left on the shelf' was the ultimate disgrace to women. But not to me. Yes, I could see how happy Mum and Dad were together, but I simply could not envisage myself entering into and sustaining a mutually favourable partnership like theirs.

I gave my all to my work, considering myself very fortunate to research, lecture and teach in such a prestigious university. I enjoyed the way my students affectionately teased me for my 'birds nest' hair, the thick glasses always perched at the end of my nose or on top of my head, my unfashionable clothes and lace-up shoes. I wore a red skirt once, a big departure from my usual black or brown, and it seemed to cause the most ridiculous ripple throughout the campus which I found baffling and embarrassing and I didn't wear it again. It was enough for me that they loved my lectures and tutorials, and I absolutely loved my life.

I was not lonely—who can be lonely surrounded by magnificent buildings, all of them steeped in history and filled with other academics and students who hung on your every word, not to mention a world-renowned library of books at one's disposal? I wished for nothing more, and that's the truth.

Of course, it's obvious that fate had other ideas, otherwise you would not exist and there would be no need for me to recount all this, which is painful for me to do. I know you must have asked yourself a thousand times how I, a frumpy thirty-something with an aversion to relationships, came to have an affair. I often wondered that myself, actually, during the time the liaison lasted. However, as I couldn't explain it even to myself, I chose to simply enjoy it, for I knew it wouldn't last.

Our first encounter was hardly an exciting one. I'd just come out of a lecture and I did not have much time before a tutorial with a very promising doctoral student, so had dashed from my office to get something to eat. When I reached the till, my tray loaded with food, I found that I had left my purse behind and so had no money to pay for my meal.

I asked for a piece of paper and a pen to write down my name and department so I could settle the debt later, and a man behind me in the queue offered to pay. I turned, expecting to see a colleague from my own department, but my eyes met those of a stranger, the bluest and most piercing eyes I had ever seen. I can only describe what I felt with a well-worn cliché: it was like being hit by a bolt of lightning. I stuttered my thanks and said I would pay him back if he would tell me which department he worked in. He shrugged that off, saying my company over lunch would be payment enough.

He proceeded to follow me over to a table with his own lunch and we sat opposite each other, me instantly forgetting that I was meant to be eating fast and running back to my rooms to prepare for my student.

That lunch was a turning point for me. I can't tell you why what subsequently happened did happen, because, as I've already said, I had no wish to have more than a professional connection with another person.

He was so much older than me, not particularly good looking apart from those eyes, but he had an intellect and charisma that was hard to ignore. He created sensations within me that I had never felt before, and I found I liked it. We talked and talked. I was late for the tutorial —for the first time ever— and I could hardly keep my mind on my work all afternoon. All I could think about was him.

Though I tried to stop, to focus on my students, I found myself constantly wondering if he was thinking of me, and that took me back to those teenage girls weeping and wailing because they'd fallen for someone and didn't know if he was interested in return. I remembered how much effort they put in to themselves to impress the opposite sex, and for the first time I looked at myself in the mirror with a critical eye, trying to see how he had viewed me.

I remembered, then, on the occasion of my sixteenth birthday, Mum asking me what I'd like for a present. I wrote out a list of textbooks, suggesting she choose one or two, and she glanced at it before saying that what she'd had in mind for me was a new outfit, or a trip to a stylist to have my hair cut. When I laughed, not for a minute thinking she was serious, tears had sprung into her eyes and she'd said with sadness and bewilderment that it was as if I went out of my way to look plain and dowdy. But it was hardly that; to say I went out of my way inferred a deliberation that simply wasn't there. I was totally unconcerned with the way I looked, wanting only to be left alone to focus on my books and, later, of teaching others who were equally keen to learn.

On this fateful day, though, I went straight to a mirror as soon as I got home. The only one I owned hung above the mantelpiece, so I had to take it down and prop it on the floor angled against the bed in order to see most of myself in its reflection.

I had always acknowledged that my dress sense was non-existent, but how I could change that I really didn't know as I simply hated shopping for clothes. I thought of my mother's colourful wardrobe, all her garments skilfully made by her own hand. The only things she spent any spare money on were shoes—she had so many pairs of shoes! I had two pairs in the same, flat-heeled style, one pair black, the other brown, three long skirts and some long, loose sweaters, in either black or brown. My few clothes took up very little space in my small apartment and it made dressing each morning quick and easy.

I hung the mirror back in its place so I could lean close and study my face without my glasses. I was nonplussed to say the least at how bright my eyes and how flushed my cheeks were, because I knew the cause was the amazing and scintillating hour I'd spent with a charming, tantalising man. Despite everything, he had somehow triggered something in me I hadn't known I possessed. But I had to admit to myself that he would have forgotten me within minutes of us parting company, for I was under no illusion that I would be of interest to a virile, dynamic man like him.

But I was wrong about that, because he did remember me!

He sought me out and in no time at all I found myself caught up in my first, my only, romantic affair. He told me straight away that he was married, but gave me what I now know to be the old line of 'my wife doesn't understand me' and I agreed to keep our liaisons secret.

I wanted it secret anyway for my own sake, not just for his or his family's, because it was all so strange, so completely alien to me, but a colleague who saw us together warned me that he was renowned for breaking hearts with his extra-marital activities. Further, she told me that she knew for sure that his wife was nothing like the uncaring woman he painted her to be; on the contrary, she was a delightful person who was very supportive of his career and seemingly oblivious to his adulterous affairs.

I'm ashamed to say I didn't want to listen. I didn't want to listen because I was in love. My body had been awakened to the point I craved his touch every minute of every day. My work suffered, I became less attentive to my students and was apt to lose the thread or wander off-topic in my lectures. The changes in me both mental and physical did not go unnoticed and inevitably we were spotted together by staff and students, so all too soon rumours about us started to fly.

That's when he started hinting that we should calm things down between us, admitting what I already knew by then, that he would never leave his wife. I knew the end was coming. If I wanted our affair to continue it would have to be entirely on his terms, namely that we would see less of each other and would have to be far more careful not to be seen together.

It became so stressful I ended it between us. I was distraught, but could see no choice. For the first time, I started to think about his family and how dishonest he must be at heart to do what he did. I threw myself back into my work, but every now and then he would call and, though I am ashamed to admit my weakness, I would allow him to come to my place. We carried on this way for too many months, with each quick, fumbling visit leaving me heartsick, guilty, and used.

And then I found out I was pregnant.

He became so cold towards me when I told him, even suggesting that he might not be the father. I remember so clearly how his eyes had turned icy and mean, and his mouth had set into a thin, angry line as a deep red flush suffused his skin, making him look ugly. He shouted that he had his reputation to think about, a wife and family he wanted to keep.

It became obvious to me, as it should have done long before, that I had never been anything more than an amusing diversion to him. My naivety had intrigued and enticed him and my slavish adoration of him had kept him coming back for more. But it had never been anything to do with love, and I was soon to learn that he already had his eye on a new PhD student. (As an aside from my own story, I'm happy to tell you that she rejected him, which hit his ego very hard. Whether it was due to the anonymous note I sent her or her own innate common sense I will never know, but I like to think I did her a favour. She went on to be a top researcher at Oxford and is often to be seen these days on quality science programmes on television!).

I know you are hoping for me to finally reveal the name of your father, but I vowed that I never would disclose his identity, not even to you. This wasn't for his sake; I did it for his family. I met his wife once, when she acted as hostess at a formal inter-departmental event. It was a shock to see how attractive she was, how relaxed in company, and I couldn't help but admire how easily she moved around the room and conversed with everyone, including me.

It was this brief meeting that finally made me realise, truly see, what an utter fool I had been. I was no longer in love with him (or maybe I should be truthful and call it lust) and in fact it shocked me to realise that I actually disliked him.

The fact remained though that I faced being a single mother at the age of thirty-nine, a full nineteen years older than Mum when she'd had me. At first, I thought I could cope, but I was soon so out of my depth, so confused by the emotional turmoil within me, that I felt the only sensible action was to take an extended leave of absence from the university, close up my apartment, and return home.

All through my pregnancy it was hard not to resent the baby I was carrying (I do not say 'you' because, of course, I did not know you), for the impact on my life seemed beyond enormous. I had been forced to take leave from the job I loved more than anything else in the world; I felt sick all day, not just in the mornings; I ballooned like a whale, not only my stomach with the normal changes of pregnancy, but my ankles, feet and fingers too. I hated the indignities of the pre-natal examinations and was terrified of the birth and what would be expected of me once I had a baby to care for, terrified that I might not be able to return to teaching and research, for how could I do that and look after a child by myself? I was so confused, so disappointed in myself, that I considered giving my baby up for adoption. Surely, I told myself, it would be the best thing, both for the baby and for myself because I was not, most emphatically not, motherly material.

Oh, the horror on Mum's face when I told her what I planned to do. She insisted that I would love you once you were born, once I had actually gazed on your face and into your trusting eyes, but I didn't believe her. As my due date got nearer we went round and round in circles, me arguing for adoption for the baby's sake as much as my own, Mum and Dad telling me it would be the biggest mistake of my life.

But when you did finally come into the world and had been placed, clean and sweet-smelling in my arms, I did love you —I do love you, with all my heart—but I still did not think I could or should keep you.

That looks so cold, written down, but it was the opposite, believe me. My thoughts went relentlessly round and round until I thought my head would explode. I found it almost impossible to feed you and I wept and wailed about my shortcomings in that most basic maternal function until I was actually sick, alarming the nurses in the maternity ward. They assured me that bottle feeding you would be fine and I shouldn't feel guilty about it, and they called Mum in to try and calm me down.

She and Dad walked in together, and I could tell immediately that they had something important to say to me. Mum picked you up out of the cot and held you so naturally, so lovingly, I saw in that moment that that was how she must have held me when I was a baby. How disappointed they must be in the way I turned out, I thought. They sat together by my bed, Mum cradling you, Dad holding out his hand so your fist could grasp his little finger, and he spoke first, clearing his throat and not quite looking at me.

"You can go back to your job at the university," he said. "And we will raise your daughter."

Mum was gazing down at you, then she looked up at me with tears in her eyes, and said, "She is our granddaughter. Our family. You can't just give her away. You can't!"

I can't tell you how happy, how relieved I was at their

decision. The thought of giving you to strangers was eating me up inside, but this glorious offer literally made the sun shine that day. I knew what wonderful parents they would be to you and I would still be able to see you, to watch you grow up.

They took us both home the next day and Mum helped me immeasurably in the first few weeks. I was baffled by your needs, struggling to keep up with the constant feeding and deal with the appalling nappies that had to be changed all too often. It didn't help that you were a screamer from the time you took your first breath! You were difficult in every respect and so hard to settle that it seemed to me that you sensed my inadequacies and were determined to drain every ounce of strength and tolerance I had.

Only my parents could soothe you, so more and more they took over the care of you, making sure that by the time I was ready to leave and return to my life in Cambridge you would not miss me.

I didn't give you a name until you were almost six weeks old. I suggested Mum decide what to call you, but she insisted that it was for me to name you.

"You are her mother," she said. "And she will be raised knowing that. You've had time with her now, so surely you have a name in mind?"

Until that moment I hadn't. You were 'the baby' but suddenly I knew what I wanted to call you: Kathleen, after Dame Kathleen Lonsdale, a heroine of mine. I know you don't care for the name, but look her up, you'll see why I admired her so.

I remember the weekends when I visited, walking into the kitchen to find you standing on a little stool, helping to make pastry for apple pies or batter for Walter's favourite pancakes. All the things you two made together would have filled a bakery shop twice over! And you loved following her as she cleaned the house, clutching your own feather duster, copying her with your toy vacuum cleaner.

You were always pleased to see me, keen to show me what you'd done at school, or what you'd baked that day with your gran, but you were like that with everybody. You seemed to instinctively know that I was not the type to get down on the floor and play at 'shop' or pretend tea parties, or want to help you delve into the dressing-up box that Verity had created for you, so you didn't ask me to join in your games. Your gran was your playmate, your confidante, the one you really loved, but I was fine with that because you and I got along well enough, considering the circumstances.

Well enough, that is, until you reached your teens and we started to clash over your future.

Of course, I rather expected you to be like me, someone who loved books and school and learning and you proved to be very clever and schoolwork was quite easy for you, so I didn't think it unreasonable to want and expect you to do well academically, go to university and get a degree.

You had your own ideas though, and the eruption that occurred when I refused to allow you to leave school before you had even sat for A-Levels is forever seared on my memory. I'd had no idea until then that you possessed such a temper! How had it happened that I had one day left a giggly, amenable little girl who loved to bake fairy cakes and returned to find a sophisticated, stubborn young woman in her place? Who was this person with beads in her hair and artfully applied make-up on her lovely young face?

I'm sure I don't need to remind you of the day we had a complete meltdown of understanding that so irreparably damaged our relationship. You started by accusing me of neglecting my maternal duties, even though you knew full well I could not have given you the blissfully happy childhood you'd had through being raised by your grandparents. You screamed that I had no right to tell you what to do, that I had forfeited any rights at all by choosing not to raise you, and although Mum tried to smooth the waters as she always did, you were having none of it.

And then you asked the question that finally broke us, the question I could not and would not answer. I can picture you now as if it were yesterday, a bundle of fury planted in front of me, hands bunched into fists, demanding to know who your father was so you could go and find him and tell him what a dreadful mother I was.

I was forced to tell you that he'd died, which is the truth, but you refused to believe me. Our long estrangement following that day hurt me badly, and I was truly sorry to come crashing back into your life the way I did when I broke my arm.

I had hoped it would bring us closer together, especially as you were missing your gran so much, but I think our individual chemistry is of the volatile kind, not at all meant to mix in the same environment. I did miss you, though, once I was home and was sad when I realised that you were happy to go back to the way things had been before.

That's why I did not contact you when I received the diagnosis that I have dementia. I had suspected it for some time, several years actually, but diagnosis can be tricky and it took a while to have it confirmed. I have researched it thoroughly and am fully cognisant of what is ahead of me. It is daunting, to say the least, but my pragmatic nature is guiding me through the things I need to do.

I write in the full awareness that the disease will progress from decision-making and day-to-day tasks becoming difficult, as they are swiftly becoming, to the point when I will be incapable of independent living. My apartment and most of my possessions will be sold and the firm managing my finances have their instructions, so there will be no financial burden on you.

I have made arrangements for admission to Rainstones House when my doctor deems it necessary, because I want to be near you at my life's end. I know full well what is ahead of me now, whether it be slow or whether it be quick, and so I know that eventually I will no longer be myself and I will no longer recognise you. It is not a future I had ever contemplated, but I doubt anyone does, do they?

If you do not visit, I hope that somewhere in my diseased brain I will remember that you live not far away, and on that one day a week when you work in the hospice wing you'll be very close indeed. It is lovely that you use your skills to ease the lives of those who are dying, and I am sorry I did not recognise this in you earlier. Maybe I will even try one of your therapies when I am there, who knows?

I believe that you will come and visit me. I like to imagine you sitting beside me, talking to me. I hope I will be compos mentis for long enough after my admission to Rainstones House to know that you come, for by the time you receive this letter I will be beyond the point of recognising anyone or anything.

I am a scientist and have never believed that there is anything such as a soul or a spirit, as you do, but now I am facing death I have read many books about dying and am giving it due consideration. If our thoughts are energy and energy cannot be destroyed, maybe the thinking part of ourselves does continue to exist when we die? It's a comforting prospect.

I want to thank you, my daughter. Thank you for not turning away from me when I broke my arm, though I would not have blamed you if you had. I am under no illusion that you found my presence in the cottage for those many weeks very demanding, but in my defence, I was already exhibiting the early symptoms of dementia.

At the very least, I can see two good things coming out of my illness. The first good thing is that it has made me want to explain myself to you, in the hope that you will finally see that what I did when you were a baby was done out of love and an honest evaluation of my own maternal shortcomings. I am sorry you resented me for it, but I think you know in your heart that you were raised by the perfect couple, Verity and Walter. The second, and more important thing, is that I have the chance to tell you what a wonderful young woman you turned out to be.

With love
Your mother xxx

THE END

About the Author

J Merrill Forrest's deep interest in the supernatural is a major theme in her writing. For more than thirty years Jane has researched her subject, visiting psychics, mediums, Spiritualist churches and séances, always keeping an open and questioning mind, hunting down evidence. At age 40, Jane followed her dream of going to university and gained a BA (Hons) in English Literature, and returned to academia ten years later to gain her MA in Creative Writing. It was during this time she began to work on her novel, 'Flight of the Kingfisher,' published in 2015, which deals with the emotive and polarising subject of life after death and introduced psychic medium Alex Kelburn. He returns in her latest novel, 'The Waiting Gate,' the main theme of which is dementia and what happens to those who 'disappear' as the disease takes hold.

Find out more at www.jmforrest.com
Follow her on Twitter: @jmerrillforrest
Facebook.com/jmerrillforrest